New Qualitative Methodologies in Health and Social Care Research

D1335243

Research is increasingly important in health and social care, and is becoming central to evidence-based practice. This edited volume brings together innovative contributions from a range of professionals and research scientists who are interested in new approaches to qualitative research in health and social care.

This book covers a range of new qualitative methodologies including discourse analysis, imagework, cut-up technique, minimalist passive interviewing technique and social action research. The histories of these new methodologies are discussed and their applicability to practice outlined. The book also explores recent developments in research and their implications for delivering good practice. The book is illustrated throughout by examples drawn from practice settings.

New Qualitative Methodologies in Health and Social Care Research aims to encourage an in-depth appreciation of the concept of 'evidence' – what it means and the consequences of it being applied. It will:

- enable professionals, academics and students to learn more about new qualitative methodologies
- broaden understanding of notions of good practice
- encourage new thinking about the application of methodologies to practice.

This book is important for anyone involved in health and social care, including practitioners, primary care professionals, social scientists and researchers. It will also be invaluable for those teaching and studying these topics.

Dr Frances Rapport is The Julian Tudor Hart Senior Research Fellow at the Primary Care Group, University of Wales, Swansea.

We are, of course, [also] well aware of the great conurbations. But not of the edgelands.

Marion Shoard, *Edgelands* (2002)

New Qualitative Methodologies in Health and Social Care Research

Edited by Frances Rapport

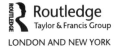

LONDON AND NEW YORK

First published 2004
by Routledge
29 West 35th Street
New York NY 10001

Simultaneously published in the UK
by Taylor & Francis
11 New Fetter Lane, London EC4P 4EE

Routledge is an imprint of the Taylor & Francis Group

Typeset in Sabon by GreenGate Publishing Services, Tonbridge, Kent
Printed and bound in Great Britain by TJ International Ltd, Padstow, Cornwall

Every effort has been made to ensure that the advice and information in this book is true and accurate at the time of going to press. However, neither the publisher nor the authors can accept any legal responsibility or liability for any errors or omissions that may be made. In the case of drug administration, any medical procedure or the use of technical equipment mentioned within this book, you are strongly advised to consult the manufacturer's guidelines.

British Library Cataloguing in Publication Data
A catalogue record for this book is available from the British Library

Library of Congress Cataloging in Publication Data
A catalog record for this book has been requested

ISBN 0-415-30564-0 (hbk)
ISBN 0-415-30565-9 (pbk)

Contents

Illustrations

Tables

Boxes

About the contributors

Contributors come from across the United Kingdom, each at the cutting edge of research using new qualitative methodologies to explore their relationship to health and social care practice and their applicability to research. Contributors are from a variety of backgrounds including: anthropology, ethics, fine art, general practice, nursing, philosophy, primary care, psychology, sociology and social work.

Information about the authors is presented in the order in which their chapters appear in the book.

Frances Rapport is Julian Tudor Hart Senior Research Fellow at the Swansea Clinical School, University of Wales, Swansea. Dr Rapport has a particular interest in comparative qualitative research methodologies, hermeneutic phenomenology and Assisted Reproductive Technology medicine. Her PhD was based on the study of women's motivation to donate eggs and used van Manen's hermeneutic phenomenological techniques.

Recent publications

2000 Maggs-Rapport, F. 'Combining methodological approaches in research: Ethnography and interpretive phenomenology', *Journal of Advanced Nursing*, 31, 1: 219–25.

2001 Maggs-Rapport, F. 'Best research practice: In pursuit of methodological rigour', *Journal of Advanced Nursing*, 35, 3: 373–83.

2002 Maggs-Rapport, F. 'Selected annotated bibliography of phenomenological sources', Seacole Research Paper 3. Mary Seacole Research Centre, De Montfort University, Leicester. ISBN 0-9539797-2-5

Lesley Griffiths is Head of the Centre for Health Economics and Policy Studies in the School of Health Science, University of Wales Swansea. Dr Griffiths has expertise in narrative, conversation analysis and discourse analysis and concentrates on the application of these techniques to health care.

Recent publications

2001 Griffiths, L. 'Categorising to exclude: The discursive construction of cases in community mental health teams', *Sociology of Health and Illness*, 23, 5: 678–700.

2003 Griffiths, L. 'Making connections: Studies of the social organisation of health-care', *Sociology of Health and Illness*, 25, 3: 1–17.

2003 Griffiths, L. and Hughes, D. 'Going public: References to the news media in NHS contract negotiations', *Sociology of Health and Illness* (forthcoming).

Glyn Elwyn is Professor of Primary Care at the Swansea Clinical School, University of Wales, Swansea. Professor Elwyn is an expert in the field of shared decision making and patient empowerment with an international reputation in the subject and has collaborated with specialists in sociolinguistics as part of an interest in narrative and discourse analysis. He continues to work closely with the Centre for Quality of Care Research at the Universities of Nijmegen and Maastricht, Netherlands.

Recent publications

2002 Elwyn, G., Edwards, A., Eccles, M. and Rovner, D. 'Decision analysis and patient care', *Lancet*, 358, 571–4.

2003 Wensing, M., Elwyn, G., Edwards, A., Vingerhoets, E. and Grol, R. 'Deconstructing patient-centred communication and uncovering shared decision making: An observational study', *BMC Medical Informatics and Decision Making*, 2, 2.

Kip Jones is an ESRC Research Fellow at the Mary Seacole Research Centre, De Montfort University, Leicester. Dr Jones has a particular interest in narrative methods and the storied nature of social health histories; his PhD explored 'narratives of identity and the informal care role'. Dr Jones has presented at a number of international conferences on the topic of narrative biography and is Associate Book Review Editor of the online journal, *Forum: Qualitative Social Research*.

Recent presentations

2001 'Non-verbal clues in narration', Centre for Biography in Social Policy, London.

2001 'Beyond the text: An Artaudian take on non-verbal clues', International Sociological Association Biography Society, Kassel, Germany.

2003 'One-day Masterclass in Narrative Interpretation', Centre for Postgraduate Studies, Swansea Clinical School, University of Swansea, Wales.

Recent publications

2004 (with E. Wu, F. Rapport & T. Greenhalgh) 'Soldiers become casualties: Doctors' accounts of the SARS epidemic', in T. Greenhalgh, B. Hurwitz & V. Skultans, eds, *Narrative Research in Health & Illness*, London: BMJ Books.

Hugh Chadderton is Consultant Nurse for Older People at the Ceredigion and Mid-Wales NHS Trust, Senior Lecturer in the School of Health Science at the University of Wales Swansea and former University of Wales and University of Wisconsin-Madison Scholar. Dr Chadderton uses Gadamerian hermeneutics to inform his work as lead clinician and named consultant for day care.

Recent publications
1998 Chadderton, H. M. 'Thinking about nursing homes', *Journal of Nursing Management*, 6, 4: 191–2.
2000 McLaughlin, F. E., Barter, M., Thomas, S. A., Rix, G., Coulter, M. and Chadderton, H. 'Perceptions of registered nurses working with assistive personnel in the United Kingdom and the United States', *International Journal of Nursing Studies*, 6: 46–57.
2003 Chadderton, H. M. 'Familiar dwelling, fractured dwelling and new dwelling: A Heideggerian–Gadamerian hermeneutic study of the Being of older people in nursing homes', unpublished PhD thesis, University of Wales College of Medicine, Cardiff.

Les Todres PhD is a clinical psychologist and Professor of Qualitative Research and Psychotherapy at the Institute of Health and Community Studies, Bournemouth University. His previous occupational roles have included head of a student counselling service and director of a clinical psychology training programme. He has also worked within NHS clinics and GP practices. He has published in the areas of phenomenological psychology and integrative psychotherapy.

Recent publications
2000 Todres, L., Fulbrook, P. and Albarran, J. 'On the receiving end: a hermeneutic–phenomenological analysis of a patient's struggle to cope while going through intensive care', *Nursing in Critical Care*, 5, 6: 227–87.
2001 Todres, L. and Wheeler, S. 'The complementarity of phenomenology, hermeneutics and existentialism as a philosophical perspective for nursing research', *International Journal of Nursing Studies*, 38: 1–8.
2002 Todres, L. 'Humanising forces: Phenomenology in science; psychotherapy in technological culture', *Indo-Pacific Journal of Phenomenology*, 3: 1–16.

Immy Holloway is Professor of Health Studies at the Institute of Health and Community Studies, Bournemouth University. Professor Holloway has been the initiator and conference coordinator on a number of national and international qualitative research conferences including the IHCS European Conference in Qualitative Health and Social Care 2002.

Recent publications
1997 Holloway, I. *Basic Concepts for Qualitative Research*, Oxford: Blackwell Science.

2000 Holloway, I. *Getting a PhD in Health and Social Care*, Oxford: Blackwell Science.
2002 Holloway, I. and Wheeler, S. *Qualitative Research in Nursing*, 2nd edn, Oxford: Blackwell Publications.

Nigel Rapport holds the Chair of Anthropological and Philosophical Studies in the Department of Social Anthropology at the University of St Andrews. He is also Professor (Adjunct) at the Norwegian University of Science and Technology, Trondheim. He has conducted participant observation research in England, Newfoundland, Israel and Scotland. His research interests in anthropology include the study of: individuality, consciousness, literary anthropology, identity, conversation analysis, violence, community studies, aesthetics, globalisation, symbolic interactionism and postmodernism.

Recent publications
2002 Rapport, N. J. and Amit, V. *The Trouble with Community: Anthropological Reflections on Movement, Identity and Collectivity*, London: Pluto Press.
2002 Rapport, N. J., ed., *British Subjects: An Anthropology of Britain*, Oxford: Berg.
2003 Rapport, N. J. *I am Dynamite: An Alternative Anthropology of Power*, London: Routledge.

Iain Edgar is a Lecturer at the Department of Anthropology, Durham University. Dr Edgar has expertise in the use and development of imagework, with particular interest in cultural approaches to dreams. He teaches human sciences modules in mental health and illness and health and society. He is writing a book on imagework as a research methodology for Routledge.

Recent publications
1998 Edgar, I. 'The Imagework Method in health and social science research', *Qualitative Health Research*, 1, 2: 192–211.
2001 Edgar, I. 'Cultural dreaming or dreaming cultures? The anthropologist and the dream', *KEA: Zeitscrift für Kulturwissenschaften* (German interdisciplinary social science journal), 13: 1–20.
2002 Edgar, I. 'Invisible elites: Authority and the dream', *Dreaming*, 12, 2: 79–92.

Francis C. Biley is Senior Lecturer at the School of Nursing, University of Wales College of Medicine, Cardiff. Dr Biley has published on a diverse range of topics and has nearly 200 papers in scientific and other nursing journals to his name. Dr Biley is particularly interested in the use of the arts and humanities in health care education and in William S. Burroughs' literary cut-up technique, which aims to enable new understandings of health care and experiences related to health care.

Recent publications

2000 Biley, F. C. 'The effects on patient well-being of music listening as a nursing intervention: A review of the literature', *Journal of Clinical Nursing*, 9: 668–77.

2001 Biley, F. C. 'Developing health care environments in order to maximise healing', in Rankin-Box, D., ed., *The Nurse's Handbook of Complementary Therapies*, 2nd edn, Edinburgh: Churchill Livingstone, pp. 223–9.

Christopher Maggs is Honorary Professor of Clinical Practice and Development, University College, Worcester and Mid Staffordshire General Hospitals NHS Trust. He has worked as a researcher in a number of fields including nursing, history and social sciences. He is clinically based and responsible for a 24-bed hospital ward, as well as being the NHS Trust Clinical Ethics Advisor. He is particularly interested in the need for rigour in research methodologies, whichever paradigm.

Recent publications

2002 Maggs, C. and Rapport, F. 'Titmuss and the gift relationship: Altruism revisited', *Journal of Advanced Nursing*, 40, 5: 495–503.

2002 Maggs, C. 'Milestones in British nursing', in Daly, J., Speedy, S., Jackson, D. and Darbyshire P., eds, *Contexts of Nursing*, Oxford: Blackwell, pp. 12–21.

2003 Maggs, C. and Coufopoulos, A. M. 'A longitudinal study of the dietary intake of 51 adolescents in South Staffordshire, UK', *International Journal of Nutrition and Education*, 40, 1: 21–6.

Jennie Fleming is a Senior Lecturer (Research) at the Centre for Social Action, De Montfort University, Leicester. For the past ten years Jennie has worked for the Centre for Social Action as a trainer, consultant and researcher working with communities to encourage participation. Her main academic interests are social action, empowerment and participation.

Recent publications

1999 Fleming, J. and Ward, D. 'Research as empowerment: The social action approach', in Shera, W. and Wells L., eds, *Empowerment Practice: Developing Richer Conceptual Foundations*, Toronto: Canadian Scholars' Press.

2000 Fleming, J. 'Action research for the development of children's services in Ukraine', in Kemshall, H. and Littlechild, M., eds, *User Involvement and Participation in Social Care: Research Informing Practice*, London: Jessica Kingsley.

2002 Fleming, J. 'Participative evaluation', in Dearling, A., ed., *Making a Difference: Practice and Planning in Working with Young People in Community Safety and Crime Prevention Programmes*, Lyme Regis: Russell House Press.

Dave Ward is Professor and Head of School in the School of Health and Applied Social Sciences, De Montfort University, Leicester. Professor Ward's main academic interest is groupwork, social action, empowerment and user involvement and he has been instrumental in the development of the self-directed learning model in groupwork with Audrey Mullender.

Recent publications
1991 Mullender, A. and Ward, D. *Self-Directed Groupwork: Users take Action for Empowerment*, London: Whiting and Birch.

1996 Ward, D., ed., *Groups and Research* (special edition of the journal *Groupwork*, 9: 2), London: Whiting and Birch.

2000 Ward, D. and Boeck, T. 'Addressing social exclusion: The social action research contribution to local development', in Matthies, A-L. Jarvela, M. and Ward, D., eds, *From Social Exclusion to Participation: Explorations Across Three European Cities*, Jyvaskyla, Finland: University of Jyvaskyla, pp. 41–60.

Preface and acknowledgements

Aim of the book

The aim of this collected volume is to better inform research and practice in health and social care by raising awareness of the potential use for new qualitative methodology and its application to practice. New qualitative methodology is discussed in terms of its history, methods and applicability to health and social care practice. In order of chapter appearance, following an introduction to new qualitative methodology (Frances Rapport), methods covered are:

Chapter 1: Discourse analysis (Griffiths and Elwyn)
Chapter 2: Biographic narrative interpretive method (Jones)
Chapter 3: Hermeneutic method (Chadderton)
Chapter 4: Descriptive phenomenological method (Todres and Holloway)
Chapter 5: Interpretative anthropological method (Nigel Rapport)
Chapter 6: Imagework (Edgar)
Chapter 7: Cut-up technique (Biley)
Chapter 8: Historiography (Maggs)
Chapter 9: Social action research (self-directed groupwork method) (Fleming and Ward)

In exploring recent developments in qualitative methodologies and their implications for, and impact on, the delivery of health and social care and the evaluation of good practice, the volume and the individual contributions will:

- broaden understanding of notions of good practice;
- enable health and social care professionals and academics to learn more about new qualitative methodologies;
- encourage an understanding of the application of methodologies to practice.

There is pressure on health and social care professionals to combine their health or social care work with research – however limited – in order to achieve 'best practice'. This is normally seen as entailing simply keeping up with the latest literature and apprehending the results of recent evidence-based research. But evidence is not so simple or transparent a concept. Evidence, in fact, is closely related to research methodology. Different methodologies can put forward different 'evidence': both different kinds of facts and, to an extent, different facts per se. There are more research methodologies and more evidences about in 'science' than many health and social care professionals may be aware.

But these other methodologies and evidences may have direct relevance for them nonetheless; becoming aware of a range of different methodologies and evidence can assist health and social care professionals in their efforts to achieve a timely best practice.

This book brings together health and social care professionals and a range of research scientists in order to explore ways in which notions of best practice can be broadened, and a diversity of methodologies and evidences brought into the world of health and social care. This will be done through an in-depth appreciation of the concept of evidence: what it means, how it is arrived at and the consequences of it being applied.

Unifying factors between chapters

The nine chapters in the book will cover a diverse range of approaches to qualitative methodology, spanning a spectrum of responses to the relationship of theory to practice. However, several factors unite them:

- interest to a range of professionals from different disciplines, making them accessible to a wide audience of health and social care professionals and academics;
- credibility, coming as they do from recognised experts in the field of health and social care research;
- understanding of complex issues presented in a clear and concise manner without misuse or inconsistency of methodological precepts;
- grasp of developments in qualitative methodology through clear demonstration of its applicability to our understanding of health organisations and practice;
- international application, since issues pertinent to methodological decision making transcend nationality.

Potential audience

This book should, therefore, appeal to health and social care practitioners, general practitioners, and primary care professionals and researchers, as well as to health and social care researchers, postgraduate and PhD students studying medicine, nursing, the social sciences and social work, lecturers in health and social care practice and research, and health services researchers.

With a desire to improve patient care delivery and work towards best practice, the volume is a timely reminder of the value of applying theory to clinical research and practice and the chapters, with their underlying methodological discussions, will have international relevance.

Acknowledgements

I would like to acknowledge the unerring support of family, friends and colleagues. I would also like to thank the contributors for their continued encouragement and belief in this project. These chapters are the result of a successful programme of seminars and masterclasses in New Qualitative Methodology, presented to packed audiences at the University of Wales Swansea over the past two years. The chapters display the breadth and diversity of the contributors' knowledge and expertise and their ability to bring creativity to their work and make it shine.

Frances Rapport
Swansea, September 2003

Foreword

> Reality is not given: it has to be continually sought out, held – I am
> tempted to say salvaged [...] Reality always lies beyond.
>
> (Berger 1984: 72)

I increasingly feel there is something impoverished, desiccated and confined
about the way in which we approach explanation and understanding within
the social sciences. We dig a hole, stick the name of a discipline or a method
on it, get into it, and talk only to those who want to get into the hole with
us; and they are only allowed in once they have learned the methodological
rules. We are ever so cautious, only making use of what can be seen from
our particular bunker. We fear using our imaginations, as if this would
somehow distort, or lead us away from, reality. But, as the great art critic
and novelist John Berger reminds us, reality is an imaginative construction.
And whether we approach reality through 'science', 'religion', 'literature' or
'history', we are imaginatively seeking something out, trying to grasp hold
of it. Of course, in this process, we need to collect evidence and develop
methods for doing so: statistics, experiments, systematic reviews, documents, talk, photographs or artefacts. But the evidence and the methods are
not the reality. Reality is the sweep of the imagination in relation to the evidence, the theories and arguments we develop for our interpretations. The
evidence does not speak for itself, and our methods are not simple windows
onto reality. Reality lies beyond and has to be salvaged.

There are many guides to how to do this well. They usually focus on a
particular method, or a class of methods. We have books on interviewing,
participant observation, ethnography, regression analysis, documents and
so on. In particular, we have books about quantitative methods and qualitative methods, and these are two deep bunkers – so deep that once you get
in it is very difficult to get out, alive. It is hard to know when this distinction first imprinted itself on human consciousness, but it is there in the
nineteenth-century debate over 'positivism', and is anticipated by the distinction, usually expressed in German, between the *Naturwissenschaften*

and the *Geisteswissenschaften* – the sciences of nature and the sciences of spirit, what we would probably nowadays call sciences and humanities, with the social sciences taking from both, in different degrees at different times. While the drawing of boundaries between qualitative and quantitative is often self-protective or self-serving and unhelpful to the development of understanding, the deeper distinction between approaches to knowledge is a powerful one, and very important for seeing that there are different ways of grasping reality, or salvaging something from it.

The point about the social sciences, broadly understood, is that they are dealing with realities that are pre-interpreted. People's experiences, words and actions are not just data, they themselves embody interpretation, struggles to get at what lies beyond the alternating regularity and disruption of everyday life. The subjects, respondents or informants of our research projects are not simply bearers of data waiting for our expertise to illuminate the meanings and interconnections that they themselves are too limited or uneducated to perceive. They are engaged in a process of theorising their own lives, and as we observe or talk to them we need to find ways of making sense of their theories in terms of our own.

We are also increasingly expected to be able to use our knowledge to inform policy and practice. There is a growing demand for evidence in many areas of social life. You need evidence to justify a new or expensive treatment for disease, you need evidence in order to go to war, and you need evidence to show that the education you are delivering is actually educating those to whom is it delivered. Although it is sometimes a long time coming, this evidence is supposed to be visible, verifiable and valid. Policies, programmes and practices have to be evidence-based. In a world driven by the demands of policy, and real-world relevance, some of the neat disciplinary boundaries come under pressure. The complex, multi-dimensional issues raised by health, crime, education and employment demand the cooperation of people from many disciplines, and this raises profound questions about how evidence is defined, data collected, interpretations elaborated.

This collection of chapters on 'new qualitative methodology' is important for a number of reasons. First, the contributors really do come from a wide range of backgrounds – different intellectual disciplines with varying relations to worlds of practice (medicine, clinical psychology, nursing) – and are committed to linking theory to practice. Second, resisting the tendency to define qualitative methods as just like quantitative methods without the numbers, they invite us to think creatively about data and method. Third, in doing this, connections are continually made between the methods and the philosophical contexts to which the methods are connected. And finally, the real difficulties of grasping the reality of experience, language and action are confronted head on, challenging us to find innovative ways of approaching the intersubjective realities of everyday life. While there is much to be applauded in the rise of evidence-based policy and practice, we should recognise, like Martha Nussbaum, that utilitarian or rational choice approaches to public policy can leave us:

> ... blind to the qualitative richness of the perceptible world; to the separateness of its people, to their inner depths, their hopes and loves and fears; blind to what it is like to live a human life and to try to endow it with a human meaning.
>
> (Nussbaum 1995: 26–7)

I think most of the contributors to this book would agree with that. Drawing on philosophy, literature and history as well as conventional social sciences, they attempt to convert their insights into practical applications for health and social care, where the pressures to do things according to the rules can be very great indeed. At a time when the strains on health and social care brought about by years of under-funding are sometimes intolerable, discussions of approaches to subjectivity may appear luxurious. I would argue, on the contrary, that the economic and political pressures on health and social care make such explorations in salvaging reality all the more vital.

Gareth Williams
School of Social Sciences, Cardiff University

References

Berger, J. (1984) *And Our Faces, My Heart, Brief as Photos*, London: Writers and Readers Publishing Co-operative Society.

Nussbaum, M. (1995) *Poetic Justice: The Literary Imagination and Public Life*, Boston: Beacon Press.

Shifting sands in qualitative methodology

Frances Rapport

New – Not existing before; ...

(The Oxford Reference Dictionary 1987: 566)

Qualitative – (*qualis* means 'whatness') asks the *ti estin* question: What is it? What is this phenomenon in its whatness?

(van Manen 1990: 33)

Methodology – [R]efers to the general principles of investigation that guide a study, based on its underlying theoretical and philosophical assumptions. These principles will dictate that certain designs and methods are appropriate, and other designs and methods inappropriate.

(Sim and Wright 2000: 7)

From traditional beginnings ...

In health and social care research, as in the social science arena, debate surrounding the methodological divide constructed between researchers concerned with statistical modelling and those concerned with social theorising is likely to run and run (Morrow 1994; Robson 2002). Researchers continue to place themselves within either positivistic or naturalistic camps, voicing the inadequacies of the opposing camp and, by so doing, perpetuating the gulf between research strategies aligned with quantitative and qualitative methods. Qualitative researchers are criticised for producing ineffective interpretations, based on researcher subjectivity (Morrow 1994). Quantitative researchers are criticised for being steeped in 'naïve objectivity' (Morrow 1994: 202), for concentrating on causal explanations and standardised outcomes, and for being ineffectual in describing social construction, cultural change or individual experience. Quantitative researchers are said to use 'a set of ad hoc procedures to define, count and analyse [its] variables' (Silverman 2000: 5). Qualitative researchers are said to be interested in the way we might go about defining, counting and analysing – whatever these terms might mean – and blame quantitative researchers for using 'the methods of everyday life, even as they claim scientific objectivity' (Silverman 2000: 5). (See Table 1 for differences between qualitative and quantitative research.)

In order to situate new qualitative methodology at a point of departure from its more traditional forebears, a brief recapitulation of its foundations and their influence on humanistic approaches to Social Action and interpretation is necessary. Giddens (1982) argues that three separate forces – positivism, functionalism and industrial society – have affected the early development of the social sciences. Positivism (a term made popular by Saint-Simon, who referred to the 'positive' data of experience as the basis for all science (Tesch 1990)) favoured the modelling of the social sciences on the natural sciences and suggested the production of a 'natural science of society' (Giddens 1982: 2). Supported by Mill and Comte, and following in the footsteps of Newton and Locke, Saint-Simon recommended the analysis of Social Action based on the analysis of physical objects in the natural sciences through the application of the universal rules of logic and laws of causality (Hekman 1984; Jackson 1994). Functionalism endorsed a direct relationship between biology and social science in order to taxonomise social phenomena (van Manen 1990) and industrial society looked to modernisation and the belief in the transformation of contemporary society through industrialisation. These three factors, or 'the orthodox consensus' of nineteenth-century and early twentieth-century social science, as they

Table 1 Differences between qualitative and quantitative research

Quantitative ('positivistic' or 'empirical–analytical')	Qualitative ('humanistic' or 'naturalistic')
Foundation of pure fact that can be turned to for questions regarding truth	Evidence is always social
Interest in controlling events	Interest in human expression and human meaning
Relationship between cause and effect	Relationship between meaning, action and behaviour
Causal relationship described in terms of observation statements, verification and prediction	Description of human action and behaviour
The social governed by rules of law-like regularity	The social structured by meanings we give to experience
Physical events and human activities that can be measured with tools designed to produce generalisable observations	Recognition of the difference between explaining physical events and human activities
No place for interpretation. Measurable hypotheses tested to improve theory	Interpretation, grounded in understanding expressed through language
Explanation through causal analysis based on invariant laws	Explanation through interpretation and description

were later known, came to be denounced as scepticism grew in social science's positivistic and functional roots and in the security of industrial society (Giddens 1982: 3).

Within the past century, the 'orthodox consensus' has been challenged by an interest in humanistic enquiry and qualitative methodology. The revolt against positivism, led by Dilthey and Schiller, was premised upon the belief that the methods for studying inanimate objects were inappropriate when it came to the study of human beings. Dilthey insisted on two distinct kinds of sciences: the *Naturwissenschaften* (the natural or physical sciences) and the *Geisteswissenschaften* (the human sciences). Following its development in the 1920s, the human sciences encouraged a commitment to subjectivity through an appreciation of the uniqueness of human experience. Its subject matter was the human world, characterised by *Geist* – 'mind, thoughts, consciousness, values, feelings, emotions, actions and purposes', finding objectification in 'languages, beliefs, arts and institutions' (van Manen 1990: 3). With the growth of popularity in the early 1960s of humanistic disciplines such as social anthropology and interpretive sociology, an interest in human experience grew to encompass associated disciplines such as psychology, history, health care and social care. Humanistic enquiry and qualitative methodology became common currency, concentrating on personal experience and the meanings we give to our 'human-ness', as opposed to the natural sciences which looked at natural events, objects of nature and behaviour patterns (Burke Drauker 1999; van Manen 1990). Qualitative researchers started experimenting with mixing methods and methodologies. They attempted to combine aspects of phenomenology (the science of experience through consciousness), hermeneutics (the science of interpretation through language), ethnography (the science of people's day-to-day experience as observed) and grounded theory (the science of theory development grounded in data), to develop theories that would support and underpin human experience (Maggs-Rapport 2000).

Whilst such experimentation was taking place, researchers described and interpreted the human condition, cultural experiences and the effects of researcher presence on the behaviour of research participant (Denzin and Lincoln 1994). Mixing methods received mixed reviews. For example, though Johnson *et al.* (2001) have condoned this approach, saying there are 'no "real" natural laws concerning socially derived knowledge and therefore no possibilities for "pure" methods of social or interpersonal sciences' (Johnson *et al.* 2001: 249), Baker *et al.* (1992) have condemned the effects of 'method slurring'. They describe it as a lack of clarity over process and research standards, saying different methodological assumptions render the combination of methods impossible. Whilst disagreements such as this persist, researchers working within humanistic paradigms search for new ground to counter what still appears to be a sense of positivistic influence over the social sciences (Giddens 1974; Murphy *et al.* 1998). Most markedly, researchers attempt to develop their expertise within one qualitative methodology, inventing a host of sub-methodologies to take an individual position forward. By so doing, the whole becomes fractured and multi-faceted. Such working practices lead to methodological fragmentation as, in an attempt to understand the theoretical nuances of a chosen methodology, researchers impose false delineations on complex ideas, leading to oversimplification and misinterpretation of concepts. Sub-methodologies in phenomenology, for example, include: philosophical phenomenology, hermeneutic phenomenology, Heideggerian phenomenology, Husserlian phenomenology, transcendental phenomenology, Gadamerian phenomenology and phenomenological philosophy, and there is mutual distancing amongst these sub-methodologies. A host of 'evidence' of the need for mutual distancing is presented to support associated positions (Giorgi 1992; Giorgi 2000a; Paley 1997) and methodological association or the strength of methodological 'wholism' is rarely discussed.

New ways of expressing the human condition

Within methodological fragmentation, exploratory, descriptive, narrative and interpretive forays into how we make sense of the human condition continue to dominate qualitative research studies. The more recent interpretive research enquiries perpetuate methodological fragmentation by concentrating on the tools of interpretation and description to the exclusion of all other aspects of a study. The methods used for data collection and analysis, the 'making sense of' data, take precedence over ethical issues and the relationship between research questions and methods (Porter 1998; Robertson-Malt 1998).

Following on from a history of qualitative methodology this section responds to a concentration on method, looking at those methods most frequently used in qualitative research studies and new methods coming to the fore.

At present, methods frequently used in qualitative research – such as interviews, participant observation and focus groups – are the more conventional according to qualitative expectations. This is due, in part, to their seemingly malleable qualities such as their adaptability to a range of research scenarios. However, though these methods are focused upon disproportionately to other aspects of a study, it is common for their presentation to be without justification as to researcher choice or research questions (Maggs-Rapport 2001). Little attention is paid to the reasoning behind a chosen method and although interviews, participant observation and focus groups may be appropriate for some research enquiries, they are not necessarily appropriate for all (Maggs-Rapport 2001). To be sure, it has been suggested that they may be restrictive or insensitive to the research enquiry in some instances (they cannot answer the question), leading to a call for new methods (Biley 1998). Using semi-structured interviews as an example, Jones (2003) suggests that over the past decade research using interviewing as the technique of data collection within the social sciences is premised on the researcher's predetermined assumptions which then become integral to the questioning process. This, Jones argues, limits the scope and depth of the enquiry (cf. Hockey 2002).

However, new methods within qualitative methodology are beginning to find cautious recognition. This book is about an in-depth exploration of the following methods and their relation to methodology: *biographic narrative interpretive method* (that asks a single, initial question to induce an extensive narrative); *hermeneutic method* (that explores the meanings we give to personal understanding of phenomena); *descriptive phenomenological method* (that concentrates on the use of descriptive text to elucidate phenomena); *interpretive anthropological method* (that gathers, through a subjective process, insights into the researcher's and and others' behaviour and routines); *cut-up technique* (exploring the random, cut-up interjections of text to re-contextualise perceptions of self and other); *discourse analysis* (the examination of the processes of communication to study language in context); *historical method* (an analytic approach to various historical sources to construct an account or 'composite portrait' of an event); *Social Action Research (the self-directed groupwork method)* (that facilitates a process of active learning, development and change in order to move towards personal empowerment) and *imagework* (the elicitation of implicit knowledge and self-identity through, for example, participants' use of artwork, gestalt, dreamwork and sculpting). Though it is not possible to define each method in any depth in the introduction, contributors will offer a thorough description in individual chapters, elucidating how each presents powerful tools for information elicitation.[1] (Also see Table 2 overleaf for categorisation of new qualitative methods.)

Practical application of new qualitative methodology

This section explores the possible practical application of new qualitative methodology in the health and social care setting, where new methods have been used in a variety of research scenarios. *The Social Action Research model* (Fleming and Ward 1999) within re-defined methodology, for example, has been employed in social care settings, schools, hospitals and community and health forums, to encourage personal empowerment whilst transforming people's practices and impacting on personal life chances. From the Social Action Research model, Mullender and Ward have developed the *self-directed groupwork method* (Mullender and Ward 1991), a particular application of the articulation of Social Action through emancipation and personal empowerment, which, in the research environment, is said to provide practical routes to social change. *Socio-linguistic analysis*

Table 2 Categorisation of new qualitative methodology

Arts-based research methods	Narrative-based research methods	Redefined research methods
Imagework	Discourse analysis	Social Action Research model (self-directed groupwork method)
Cut-up technique	Biographical narrative method	Interpretive anthropological method
Hermeneutic photography	Discursive narrative method	Descriptive phenomenological method
Emotion work	Socio-linguistic analysis	Hermeneutic method
Photo elicitation	Personal narrative method	
Narrative picturing	Historiography	
Vignette technique		
Dreamwork		
Performative inquiry		
Receptive and active imagery method		

(see Jordens *et al.* 2001), a method within narrative-based methodology, has been used in cancer research settings to analyse narratives of cancer and the *discursive narrative method* (see Wilkinson and Kitzinger 2000), also found within narrative-based methodology, has been used to encourage patients to think positively about cancer whilst enabling researchers to explore the content and context of patients' talk. In arts-based research methodology, emotion work (see Exley and Letherby 2001) has been used with the infertile and involuntary childless to explore lifecourse disruption; photo elicitation (see Häggström *et al.* 1994) has been used to explore the experience of living with stroke sequelae; and hermeneutic photography (see Hagedorn 1994) has been used to explore families' experiences of living with chronic illness. It would appear that for those who choose new qualitative methodologies, potential research settings are numerous (Biley 1998; Greenhalgh and Hurwitz 1998; Edgar 1999).

New qualitative research methodologies in this collection

A variety of narrative-based and arts-based and re-defined research methods are presented here in this collection. Amongst the arts-based methods, in Chapter 6, *imagework* (Edgar 1999: 199) is described as having the ability to elicit implicit knowledge and self-identities of respondents in a way that other methods cannot – a quality that is capable of affecting a positive change in our understanding of self and other, and in Chapter 7, *cut-up technique* is described as the manipulation of text to allow researchers to access different levels of understanding (also see Biley 1998). Inspired by the work of William S. Burroughs, cut-up technique alters the structure of language by creating randomly selected sentences that are 'incapable of formulation' (Biley 2000: 68, citing Burroughs 1979: 3). With no recognised point of reference, the mixing of words and sentences enables the researcher's range of vision to constantly expand, thus manifesting 'elements of non-linearity' to show 'the emergence of hidden associations and meanings' for the researcher (Biley 1998).

Amongst the narrative-based research methods presented here, *biographic narrative interpretive method* has been said to encourage the establishment of a special rapport between interviewer and interviewee (cf. Jones 2001), and in a recent exposition of this method, Jones (2003) highlights the shift created in the balance between researcher-as-investigator and researcher-as-reflective/passive-participant, within the interview scenario. In Chapter 2, Jones, citing Chamberlayne and King (2000), describes the method as 'dynamic and interpretive … with an emphasis on action and latent meaning, which distinguishes it within the broad and rich range of life history, oral history and narrative approaches'. *Discourse analysis*, discussed here in Chapter 1 by Griffiths and Elwyn, has sometimes been referred to as the analysis of language 'beyond the sentence' (Tannen 2002). Elwyn and Gwyn (1999) previously called it the study of 'language in context' (1999: 186), encouraging in-depth exploration of the process of communication when the tools normally used to examine communication are insufficient for understanding 'the layers of meaning that lie within the text of exchange' (1999: 186). Unlike some of the lesser-known 'new' methods, discourse analysis is already well recognised as an excellent technique for exploring communication within the clinician's practice. (See also Scheff (1990) who discusses discourse analysis for doctor–patient interaction.) In Elwyn and Gwyn's 1999 paper on the analysis of talk in clinical practice, the method is valued as enabling health practitioners to listen more constructively to patients' stories. Similarly, in a recent conference presentation on the use of discourse analysis in social care, Hall (2002) has described the method as offering insights into the development of policy and practice. In exploring the analysis of talk and interaction in health and social care encounters between professionals and clients, Hall (2002) suggests that discourse analysis, far from undermining professionals and professional practice, promotes communication skills through the separation of analytic insight and professional judgement.

The three strands of new qualitative methodology

These, then, are some of the methods presented in this book, which can be described collectively as 'new qualitative methodologies'. New qualitative methodologies are predominantly three interlocking strands that together cover all the qualitative methodologies. The three strands are: arts-based research, within which you will find *imagework* (Chapter 6, Edgar) and *cut-up technique* (Chapter 7, Biley); narrative-based research methodology, within which you will find *discourse analysis* (Chapter 1, Griffiths and Elwyn), *biographic narrative interpretive method* (Chapter 2, Jones) and *historic method* or *'historiography'* (Chapter 8, Maggs); and redefined methodology, within which you will find *hermeneutic method* (Chapter 3, Chadderton), *descriptive phenomenological method* (Chapter 4, Todres and Holloway), *interpretative anthropological method* (Chapter 5, Rapport) and the *Social Action Research model* (*self-directed groupwork method*) (Chapter 9, Fleming and Ward). Let us now consider each strand in turn.

Arts-based methodology

Arts-based methodology differs most from narrative-based methodology and redefined methodology in its emphasis on senses other than the verbal – most noticeably the visual. As such, it is able to express the need to over-come logocentrism (concentration on speech), through an appreciation of our multi-sensory experience of life. As with narrative-based methodology and redefined methodology, arts-based methodology links back to Dilthey's ideas about the *Geisteswissenschaften*. It concentrates on our understand-ing of the world from a participant's perspective, which is considered both unique and particular. It recognises that people act according to their own individual views and that complex behaviours cannot be explored without looking for new ways of making sense of that uniqueness.

   Imagework (Edgar 1999; Edgar 2000; Edgar 2002), *dreamwork* (LeVine 1981; Wunder 1993; Edgar 2000), *emotion work* (Exley and Letherby 2001), *performative inquiry* (Fels and Meyer 1997), *hermeneutic photogra-phy* (Hagedorn 1994), *photo-elicitation* (Radley and Taylor 2002), *receptive and active imagery method* (Dossey 1995), *cut-up technique* (Biley 1998, 1999), *vignette technique* (Finch 1987) and *narrative picturing* (Stuhlmiller and Thorsen 1997) are some of the arts-based research meth-ods currently in use in humanistic research, and within these there are data collection and analysis techniques held in common. Vignette technique, nar-rative picturing and hermeneutic photography, for example, all use displacement techniques to explore people's experiences and opinions. Visual aids are employed to remove attention from the research participant onto an unknown other. Aids include artefacts, photographs and videos, written stories and biographical narratives. Vignette technique uses the short written story as its aid. Stories are usually based on hypothetical characters in specified circumstances that can be presented as visual stimuli or read out to participants. Stories are intended to mimic or contradict the participant's own experience in order to stimulate a response. Participants may decide to place themselves within the story, or purposefully remove themselves from the story to offer an outsider perspective. Participant responses, which can be presented in a variety of ways, are said to affect 'a breaking away from the limitations imposed by personal experience and circumstances' (Finch 1987: 110).

Vignette technique and other methods that use displacement techniques are particularly useful when interviews or surveys appear threatening, morally distasteful or emotionally loaded (Finch 1987). But arts-based research methods such as vignette technique should not simply be seen as adjuncts to more traditional data collection methods, or ploys to elicit data in different ways by stimulating exciting and unpredictable responses. Rather, they offer researchers new dimensions from which to view the world. They attempt to visually recreate the research participant's world and are dependent on the sensory and the emotive. By creating a visual world, they enable people to express experiences of health and social care that may otherwise be overlooked (for example, they may reflect the child's experience of being ill). At the same time, they encourage the creator – the photographer, painter, researcher, subject, child – to present their relationship to the world in a very particular way, a relationship that, according to Sontag (1977: 4), is the closest we get to something 'that feels like knowledge'.

Narrative-based methodology

Biographical narrative interpretive method (Jones 2001; Jones 2003), *discourse analysis* (Elwyn 1997; Elwyn and Gwyn 1999), *socio-linguistic analysis* (Jordens *et al.* 2001), *personal narrative* (Riessman 1993; Frank 2001), *historiography* (Brieger 1993; Maggs, Chapter 8) and *discursive narrative method* (Wilkinson and Kitzinger 2000) are some of the methods currently in use in narrative-based methodology.

As with arts-based methodology, narrative-based methodology concentrates on the telling of stories that, through their narration, offer added meaning to both storyteller and listener. However, unlike arts-based methodology, narrative-based methodology concentrates on the verbal, the *logos*, as key to understanding. Narrative-based methodology considers the story as telling of actions and events in others' lives that encourage reflection and self-understanding for the narrator. Frank (2001) describes a world that is narratable, a world that, as we attempt to make sense of it through the stories we tell, is given form and coherence. The construction of stories takes place through the process of talking and listening (Frank 2001), for stories necessitate being heard as much as they necessitate being told. Through telling and listening, meaning is produced. For the listener, the telling of the story encourages the recording and interpretation of the storyteller's narration – in itself a representation of experience already predefined by the storyteller. Prior interpretation allows thoughts and feelings to be transformed into words and, from this position, to be interpreted into meaningful events.

As a narrative researcher, the participant's story can be considered on a number of levels: contextually (aspects surrounding the event being described), mantically (the emotions expressed) and semantically (the events as portrayed by the storyteller) (van Manen 1990). Stories can be considered linguistically (the ordering of words and sentences and the use of emphasis and pauses), historically (in temporal or spacial terms), culturally (according to ethnic or social grouping) or biographically (life stories). Thus narrative-based methodology affords us the opportunity of making sense, not only of the stories being told, but also of the presentation style, environment and culture of the narrator (Greenhalgh and Hurwitz 1998).

Personal narrative method has been used to explore illness pathways, communication between clinicians and patients, social anxiety and cultural mores (Frank 2001). The teller discusses life experiences, biographical accounts or illness events with the listener, often through informal talks that may turn into lengthy conversations. In the case of the recounting of illness events, the telling encourages a reordering of experience such as the medical examination. The examination, we are told, may initially lead to a strong sense of personal chaos or 'disembodiment', but reordering can perhaps present it as a calmer experience (Riessman 1990; Reissman 1993). In the case of the disruption of chronic illness, says Riessman (1993), reordering of events can enable the teller to reconstruct a coherent self in narratives (Riessman 1993).[2]

According to Launer (2002) and Greenhalgh and Hurwitz (1998), in the past ten years the narrative paradigm has revolutionised the thinking of many health professionals. Launer (2002) remarks that narratives have led health professionals to:

- question some of the apparently solid certainties of science and of medicine
- become more aware of their social and political roles and to examine the power relations in their encounters with patients and teams
- enrich their work by drawing their attention to the variety of cultures and beliefs with which they come into contact
- let go of a constant sense of responsibility for other people's problems and to acquire a greater sense of the possibilities open to their patients.

(Launer 2002: 1)

Launer (2002) says the turn to narrative in primary care is the result of a variety of influences: 'feminism, anti-racism, cultural studies, social sciences, post modernistic thought' (Launer 2002: 1), and that narrative-based research has encouraged clinicians to 'move away from "normative" ways of understanding people to "narrative" ones'. Jones (2003: 60) continues this line of thought, saying narrative-based research has allowed an interest in biography to develop 'as a method of knowing persons' (Jones 2003: 60). Citing Chamberlayne and King (2000: 9), Jones describes the change as 'ground-breaking' and puts its rising popularity down to researchers' 'aptness for exploring subjective and cultural formations, and tracing interconnections between the personal and the social' (2003: 60).

Redefined methodology

Self-directed groupwork method, hermeneutic method, descriptive phenomenological method and *interpretive anthropological method* are just some of the methods that fit within the overarching title of redefined methodology. Though long-standing, these methods are clearly pushing the boundaries of health and social care research forward through their ability to continually redefine themselves and, by so doing, to redefine the concepts upon which research studies are grounded. They are methods we might well recognise but for the fact that their features are rearranging through ongoing experimentation and theoretical development. According to Todres and Wheeler, in a 2001 paper exploring the 'complementarity' of phenomenology, hermeneutics and existentialism, progressive methodologies are always 'on the way' (2001: 4). They do not stop and their positions cannot be fixed because the research context, participant and researcher are always changing and adapting. Consequently, they are open to the possibility of multiple interpretations and multiple expressions, which, though lacking in uniformity and constraint, identify them as a coherent group. Interpretive anthropology, for example, has the aspiration to be in constant flux, as Rapport describes in his essay on 'methodological eclecticism' (see Rapport and Overing 2000: 245–9), and would call into question disciplinary knowledge and 'conventional and disciplinary divisions' (Rapport, Chapter 5). Interpretive anthropology lends itself to 'the narrative nature of our human-being-in-the-world, and a coming to terms with knowledge-processes which are constructive and interpretational' (Rapport, Chapter 5). As Rapport recalls in this book, what makes interpretive anthropology dynamic in its development is its recognition of the reflexive nature of the human condition: the way our consciousness of ourselves and our worlds is in constant dialectical interplay with the nature of self and world, and its openness to human imagination – 'imaginative knowing' – as its primary tool (Rapport, Chapter 5). Complexity and ambiguity are embraced in an imaginative vision, whilst the anthropologist refuses 'to be bound or restricted by the preconceptions of categorial knowledge' (Rapport, Chapter 5). It is this sense of moving methodological boundaries forward that permeates a reflexive anthropology, as it does a reflexive hermeneutics or a reflexive phenomenology. The process by which data supplied by anthropology, hermeneutics or phenomenology feeds back into society is reflexive. Reflexive enquiry, as Chadderton highlights in his chapter on hermeneutics (Chapter 3), is much aided by an appreciation of the 'connecting conversations' within the text – the way in which the hermeneutic story unfolds through a number of anchor points, commonly: the data itself, the philosophical underpinnings, other related literature and recommendations for future research or practice.

Redefined methodology is unyielding in its aspiration to lead the researcher and reader through a reflexive enquiry into 'as complex an appreciation of experience as possible' (Rapport, Chapter 5). Not for redefined methodology the step-by-step approach to method development, but rather a pursuit of the most appropriate ways to answer research questions, unrestricted by dogma and predefined structure. Structure is self-imposed by the reflexive researcher as the research study develops in an inductive, intuitive, long-term process, and the researcher is responsible for an appropriate response to the unfolding study.

Hermeneutic method and descriptive phenomenological method, as they struggle to reinterpret and re-establish a legitimate position within modern-day health and social care research, are particularly noted for their close links and their ability to support each other even though each develops differently. Indeed, it is suggested that each would lose something without the support of the other (Todres and Wheeler 2001) and that we should recognise their complementary qualities – the grounding of the research enquiry ('the *what* of our reflections' (2001: 6)), the reflexivity of the research question (steeped in our culture and history) and the humanisation of our enquiry (the expression of what it means to be human through the vehicle of common language). For Todres and Wheeler, 'hermeneutics without phenomenology can become excessively relativisitic. Phenomenology without hermeneutics can become shallow' (2001: 6).

Moving away from conventional research methods

This section considers the need to move away from conventional research methods. It is interesting to note that in spite of a plethora of work claiming qualitative methodology as its source of data, criticisms continue to rain over the lack of scientific rigour in qualitative research (Maggs-Rapport 2001; Giorgi 2000a; Giorgi 2000b). Qualitative researchers are accused of producing data that cannot be validated, results that cannot be transferred to other settings and findings that cannot be generalisable (Maggs-Rapport 2001). Researchers from within health care settings, aware of these criticisms, spend much time attempting to validate their research by supporting the transference of data to other settings and the generalisability of findings.[3] In addition to a marked concentration on data collection and analysis and a concentration on 'conventional' methods of data collection, researchers associate the validity of data with member checking (returning to participants for confirmation of data), triangulation (bringing relationships of different data sets to bear on each other), 'insider–outsider' articulation of concepts (using the views of those both more and less familiar with the research) and 'formal–informal' group analysis (Denzin 1978; Lincoln and Guba 1985; van Manen 1990). Yet validity is rarely discussed in terms of the relevance of the methodology to the chosen research question and the relationship between the research aims and objectives to methodological choices (Maggs-Rapport 2001). Whilst researchers continue to look for validity through group analysis, individual responsibility for data becomes undermined by the need to arrive at a consensus of opinion. Furthermore, consensus of opinion takes precedence over strength of individual perspective, and the desire to arrive at a 'moment of truth' becomes more important than 'journeying towards' possible truths. By building rigid frameworks around the discovery of results and the interpretation of findings, there is little room for the unexpected to happen, fresh insights to be acquired, novel understandings to be achieved or new explanatory frameworks to be developed.

It is this rigidity that highlights the major difference between conventional methods and their less conventional counterparts. The development of new qualitative methods, underpinned by new methodologies, encourages the retention of a sense of the 'unknown'. Researchers within new qualitative methodology hold an interest in the process of discovery and are prepared to take first-hand responsibility for the research findings and subsequent conclusions, irrespective of the group. The need to arrive at a conclusive endpoint is secondary to the process of discovery and leaving nothing to chance is seen as counter-productive, reducing the creative spirit and weakening the process. Leaving nothing to chance undermines the challenge of the unexpected.

What these chapters have in common is an ability to speak to the lack of conventionality in method development and usage. They are underpinned by strong methodological frameworks and emphasise the need to move away from traditional methods, highlighting the merits of diversity whilst reminding us that there are many ways of exploring the human condition (Biley 1998). These chapters are testimony to new ways of looking and the richness of lateral thinking. What holds them together is not that they all talk to new qualitative methodology, though indeed they do, but that they revisit and challenge our expectations of the process of research. Though they continue to ascribe to the rigours of a well-planned and well-executed research study, they bear witness to shifting sands in qualitative methodology.

Notes

1 *Photo elicitation technique* has recently come to prominence for its use alongside
   patient interviewing. It has been put to good purpose in exploring the patient
   experience of care (Radley and Taylor 2002) in a recent study of patients working with researchers to make sense of the hospital setting. Researchers used
   photographs, written narratives and patient interviews to examine the part the
   physical setting played in their recovery in a rehabilitation ward (Radley and
   Taylor 2002). It was found that photographs helped stimulate discussion of
   patient narratives, acting as a vehicle for accounts of experience that could be
   'routed through the image'. Photographs stood as 'triggers for memory' (Radley
   and Taylor 2002: 79). However, these techniques have also been described as
   much more than vehicles for the contextualisation of thought, offering 'direct
   entry into [their] point of view' (2002: 79). They may add a specific visual perspective on the world and can open up situations for political
   consciousness-raising. Radley and Taylor (2002) have remarked that by offering
   patients the opportunity to control the editing process, photographs can reveal
   patients' experiences of recuperation with thoughts and feelings made visible,
   thus encouraging patients to 'envision the ward setting as an imagined space'
   (2002: 80).
2 Contrary to Riessman, who considers personal narratives as data to be made
   sense of by the researcher, Frank (2001) sees narratives as not needing to be
   'made sense of' for they offer their own sense of meaning. Rather, the analysis of
   personal narrative, says Frank (2001: 1), demands a middle ground between the
   recording of a story and the drawing of 'an absolute line between knowledge
   expressed in people's stories and social scientific knowledge based on narratives
   interpreted as data'.
3 It should be noted that not all qualitative researchers respond or work in this way,
   and would consider the nature of validation, replication and generalisation in
   human experience to be part of what qualitative research sets out to explore –
   taking nothing for granted.

References

Baker, C., Wuest, J. and Stern, P. N. (1992) 'Method slurring: The grounded theory/
   phenomenology example', *Journal of Advanced Nursing*, 17, 1355–60.
Biley, F. C. (1998) 'An experiment in accessing pandimensionality: The literary poet-
   ics and deconstruction techniques of William S. Burroughs applied to the Science
   of Unitary Human Beings', Seventh Rogerian conference, Nursing and the
   Changing Person-Environment, New York University, 19–21 June.
Biley, F. C. (1999) 'The literary poetics of experience: A postmodern perspective',
   Sigma Theta Tau conference, Varying Perspectives on Post-Modernism, City
   University, London, 27 September.
Biley, F. C. (2000) 'Tracey's story and the postmodern literary poetics of experience:
   Developing a new methodology for Rogerian Science', *Visions: The Journal of
   Rogerian Nursing Science*, 8, 1, 68–73.
Brieger, G. (1993) 'The historiography of medicine', in *Companion Encyclopedia of
   the History of Medicine*, London: Routledge.
Burke Drauker, C. (1999) 'The critique of Heideggerian hermeneutical nursing
   research', *Journal of Advanced Nursing*, 30, 2, 360–73.

Burroughs, W. S. (1979) 'Electronic evolution', in *Ah Pook is Here and Other Texts*, London: John Calder.

Chamberlayne, P. and King, A. (2000) *Cultures of Care: Biographies of Carers in Britain and the Two Germanies*, Bristol: Policy Press.

Denzin, N. K. (1978) *The Research Act: A Theoretical Introduction to Sociological Methods*, New York: McGraw Hill.

Denzin, N. K. and Lincoln, Y., eds (1994) *Handbook of Qualitative Research*, Thousand Oaks, CA: Sage Publications.

Dossey, B. (1995) 'Using imagery to help your patient heal', *AJN*, June.

Edgar, I. (1999) 'The imagework method in health and social science research', *Qualitative Health Research*, 9, 2, 198–211.

Edgar, I. (2000) 'Cultural dreaming or dreaming cultures? The anthropologist and the dream', *Kea*, 13, 1–20.

Edgar, I. (2002) 'Invisible elites? Authority and the dream', *Dreaming*, 12, 2, 79–91.

Elwyn, G. (1997) 'So many precious stories: A reflective narrative of patient based medicine in general practice, Christmas 1996', *British Medical Journal*, 315, 1659–63.

Elwyn, G. and Gwyn, R. (1999) 'Stories we hear and stories we tell: Analysing talk in clinical practice, *British Medical Journal*, 318, 186–8.

Exley, C. and Letherby, G. (2001) 'Managing a disrupted lifecourse: Issues of identity and emotion work', *Health*, 5, 1, 112–32.

Fels, L. and Meyer, K. (1997) 'On the edge of chaos: Co-evolving world(s) of drama and science', *Teaching Education*, 9, 1, 75–81.

Finch, J. (1987) 'The vignette technique in survey research', *Sociology*, 21, 1, 105–14.

Fleming, J. and Ward, D. (1999) 'Research as empowerment: The Social Action approach', in Shera, W. and Wells, L. M., eds, *Empowerment Practice in Social Work*, pp. 370–89, Toronto: Canadian Scholars Press.

Frank, A. (2001) 'The politics of authenticity', Advances in Qualitative Methods conference, Institute for Qualitative Methodology, Edmonton, Alberta, 23 February.

Giddens, A. (1974) 'Introduction', in Giddens, A., ed., *Positivism and Sociology*, London: Heinemann Educational.

Giddens, A. (1982) *Profiles and Critiques in Social Theory*, London: Macmillan Press.

Giorgi, A. (1992) 'Description versus interpretation: Competing alternative strategies for qualitative research', *Journal of Phenomenological Psychology*, 23, 2, 119–35.

Giorgi, A. (2000a) 'The status of Husserlian phenomenology in caring research', *Scandinavian Journal of Caring Science*, 14, 3–10.

Giorgi, A. (2000b) 'Concerning the application of phenomenology to caring research', *Scandinavian Journal of Caring Science*, 14, 11–15.

Greenhalgh, T. and Hurwitz, B., eds (1998) *Narrative Based Medicine: Dialogue and Discourse in Clinical Practice*, London: BMJ Books.

Hagedorn, M. (1994) 'Hermeneutic photography: An innovative esthetic technique for generating data in nursing research', *Advanced Nursing Science*, 17, 1, 44–50.

Häggström, T., Axelsson, K. and Norberg, A. (1994) 'The experience of living with stroke sequelae illuminated by means of stories and metaphors', *Qualitative Health Research*, 4, 3, 321–37.

Hall, C. (2002) 'Now you're talking: Using discourse analysis in health and social care research', Qualitative Research in Health and Social Care conference, Institute of Health and Community Studies, Bournemouth, 10 September.

Hawkins, J. and Le Roux, S., eds (1987) *The Oxford Reference Dictionary*, London: Guild Publishing.

Hekman, S. (1984) 'Action as a text: Gadamer's hermeneutics and the social scientific analysis of action', *Journal for the Theory of Social Behaviour*, 14, 3, 333–54.

Hockey, J. (2002) 'Interviews as ethnography? Disembodied social interaction in Britain', in Rapport, N., ed., *British Subjects: An Anthropological Britain*, Oxford: Berg.

Jackson, W. (1994) *Methods: Doing Social Research*, Ontario: Prentice-Hall.

Johnson, M., Long, T. and White, A. (2001) 'Arguments for "British Pluralism" in qualitative health research', *Journal of Advanced Nursing*, 33, 2, 243–9.

Jones, K. (2001) 'Beyond the text: An Artaudian take on the non-verbal clues revealed within the biographical narrative process', International Sociological Association (ISA) international conference, Kassel, Germany, 25 May.

Jones, K. (2003) 'The turn to a narrative knowing of persons: One method explored', *Nursing Times Research*, 8, 1, 60–71.

Jordens, C. F. C., Little, M., Paul, K. and Sayers, E-J. (2001) 'Life disruption and generic complexity: A social linguistic analysis of narratives of cancer illness', *Social Science & Medicine*, 53, 1227–36.

Launer, J. (2002) 'Narrative based medicine: A new paradigm for primary care', Health Communication Workshop, Health Cardiff Communication Research Centre, Cardiff, 1 May.

LeVine, S. (1981) 'Dreams of the informant about the researcher: Some difficulties inherent in the research relationship', *Ethos*, 9, 4, 276–93.

Lincoln, Y. S. and Guba, E. G. (1985) *Naturalistic Inquiry*, London: Sage Publications.

Maggs-Rapport, F. (2000) 'Combining methodological approaches in research: Ethnography and interpretive phenomenology', *Journal of Advanced Nursing*, 31, 1, 219–25.

Maggs-Rapport, F. (2001) 'Best research practice: In pursuit of methodological rigour', *Journal of Advanced Nursing*, 35, 3, 373–83.

Morrow, R. A. (1994) *Critical Theory and Methodology*, London: Sage Publications.

Mullender, A. and Ward, D. (1991) *Self-directed Groupwork: Users Take Action for Empowerment*, London: Whiting and Birch.

Murphy, E., Dingwall, R., Greatbatch, D., Parker, S. and Watson, P. (1998) 'Qualitative research methods in health technology assessment: A review of the literature', *Health Technology Assessment*, 2, 16.

Paley, J. (1997) 'Husserl, phenomenology and nursing', *Journal of Advanced Nursing*, 26, 187–93.

Porter, E. J. (1998) 'On "being inspired" by Husserl's phenomenology: Reflections on Omery's exposition of phenomenology as a method of nursing research', *Advanced Nursing Science*, 21, 1, 16–28.

Radley, A. and Taylor, D. (2002) 'Images of recovery: A photo-elicitation study on the hospital ward', *Qualitative Health Research*, 13, 1, 77–99.

Rapport, N. and Overing, J. (2000) *Social and Cultural Anthropology: The Key Concepts*, London: Routledge.

Riessman, C. K. (1990) 'Strategic uses of narrative in the presentation of self and illness', *Social Science and Medicine*, 30, 11, 1195–1200.

Riessman, C. K. (1993) *Narrative Analysis*, Newbury Park, CA: Sage Publications.

Robertson-Malt, S. (1998) 'Listening to them and reading me: A hermeneutic approach to understanding the experience of illness', *Journal of Advanced Nursing*, 29, 2, 290–7.

Robson, C. (2002) *Real World Research*, Oxford: Blackwell.

Scheff, T. (1990) *Microsociology: Discourse, Emotion and Social Structure*, Chicago: University of Chicago Press.

Silverman, D. (2000) *Doing Qualitative Research*, London: Sage Publications.

Sim, J. and Wright, C. (2000) *Research in Health Care: Concepts, Designs and Methods*, Cheltenham, Glos.: Stanley Thornes.

Sontag, S. (1977) *On Photography*, New York: Noonday Press.

Stuhlmiller, C. M. and Thorsen, R. (1997) 'Narrative picturing: A new strategy for qualitative data collection', *Qualitative Health Research*, 7, 1, 140–49.

Tannen, D. (2002) 'Discourse analysis'. Available at: http://www.Isadc.org/web2/discourse.html.

Tesch, R. (1990) *Qualitative Research: Analysis Types and Software Tools*, Basingstoke, Hants.: Falmer Press.

Todres, L. and Wheeler, S. (2001) 'The complementarity of phenomenology, hermeneutics and existentialism as a philosophical perspective for nursing research', *International Journal of Nursing Studies*, 38, 1–8.

van Manen, M. (1990) *Researching Lived Experience, Human Science for an Action Sensitive Pedagogy*, Albany, NY: State University of New York Press.

Wilkinson, S. and Kitzinger, C. (2000) 'Thinking differently about thinking positive: A discursive approach to cancer patients' talk', *Social Science & Medicine*, 50, 797–811.

Wunder, D. (1993) 'Dreams as empirical data: Siblings' dreams and fantasies about their disabled sisters and brothers', *Symbolic Interaction*, 16, 2, 117–27.

Chapter 1

Discourse analysis

Addressing the communication strategies of healthcare professionals

Lesley Griffiths and Glyn Elwyn

In addition to describing discourse analysis (DA) and its use, we wish to suggest additional applications for the techniques it employs. To date, the method has focused on understanding discourse at a research level and we suggest a significant potential for the technique in the field of communication skill development, albeit with substantial modification. Can the use of analytic methods be adapted so that clinical practitioners can reflect on their own communicative practice and learn to modify their communication style? There are certainly developments being reported that should alert us to the pragmatic use of DA in this way, which we will return to at the end of the chapter (Rollnick *et al.* 2002a; Rollnick *et al.* 2002b).

Research into the communication skills of health professionals started in earnest when it became possible to record consultations. The pioneering work of Byrne and Long in general practice is testament to the approach made possible by the use of the technology as they coded and categorised hundreds of audiotapes, and published their six-stage schema of the primary care consultation (Byrne and Long 1976). For almost 30 years, variations on this 'code-category' approach have been the norm for research into health communication. Some systems take the approach of coding very short segments of speech: the most frequently used is the Roter interaction analysis system (Roter 1991; Stewart *et al.* 1995). There is definite interest in this field: a recent review of instruments revealed the existence of over 80 different scales that have been developed to date (Boon and Stewart 1998), and there can be no doubt that the research output has changed the approach to the teaching and development of communication skills in medicine (Kurtz *et al.* 1998). There have, however, been significant critiques of such a code-category approach to the understanding of human interaction, which in sum state that an analytical analysis of an aggregation of fragments cannot provide a meaningful assessment of the communication event as an entity (Inui and Carter 1985). Human interactions are subtler than a collection of phrases, however skilfully coded. It is of interest, therefore, that another approach has begun to make its presence felt in the analysis of communication between health professionals and patients: a qualitative assessment based on a detailed analysis of the content and mechanics of the talk. We refer to this as *discourse analysis* (Nessa and Malterud 1990; Waitzkin 1990).

This chapter offers an introduction to methods of language analysis that are typically clustered under the broad heading of discourse analysis. Communicating competently is an essential set of social skills which we acquire as we become members of society. The complexity of this enterprise is invisible to those who achieve competence by normal developmental pathways. In order to enhance our communication performance, it is helpful to elaborate the intricacies and analyse in more detail just what we do in talk. It is impossible to cover the debates, and the breadth and depth of the extensive literature that surrounds this area, but we shall try to provide an illustration of how it can be useful as a way of developing the communication skills of healthcare professionals. The chapter is structured in the following way:

- a brief introduction to the DA approach;
- a description of DA;
- some central features illustrated in selected extracts;
- sample analysis;
- conclusion and implications for future work.

Discourse analysis: what the approach entails

Discourse analysis is an approach to analysing talk and texts as social actions. This approach is contrasted with approaches that treat talk as reflective of a particular reality or as a channel to an underlying reality. For the purposes of discourse analysis, talk itself (and its written form, text) is the focus of attention. The attention is detailed, careful, critical and cumulative. Discourse analysts ensure that they are aware of and frequently review the work of others in the same field, in order to develop insights that may be derived from other work that appears to have only a slight or tangential relevance to the work in hand (Drew and Heritage 1992; Wooffitt 1992; Harre and Stearns 1995). Many discourse analysts also draw on the insights of those working in the area of conversation analysis, the empirical study of talk inspired by the work of Harvey Sacks (Sacks 1989; Sacks 1992).

Talk as it happens in real life ('naturally occurring' talk) provides the raw material for discourse analysts. Talk as it is generated is too rapid and complex in its construction for a detailed comparative analysis capable of revealing patterns and exceptions. For this reason talk has to be converted into a form that can be studied in detail, typically by tape recording and transcription. 'Reduced' is an apt phrase here, as it is impossible to capture the full complexity and richness of talk by transcription, however detailed the method. However, done in an expert manner, the process can preserve

many characteristics of naturally occurring talk by incorporating information about pauses, emphasis, timing and interruption using standardised
forms of notation (see Box 1.1). As far as possible, researchers seek to share
notational formats in order to compare examples of talk. Those who wish to
learn more about these processes are advised to consult other sources (Potter
1996; Edwards 1997).

The first stage of the analysis process is to collect data. Care needs to be
taken to ensure appropriate access and consent. These are significant issues
that are outside the scope of this chapter, but are critically important if you
are to engage in studies of talk. The consultations examined here are from
general medical practice in a UK setting. The consultations were tape
recorded with the consent of both participants. Both authors studied the
transcript independently, in conjunction with the tape recording of the consultation. As a preparation for more sophisticated analysis, it is best to start
by describing in everyday terms some of the most distinct characteristics of
a transcript.

In our case, we see an example of institutional talk that assumes a particular type of relationship between the speakers. We know that there is a set
of expectations that tells us something about what a consultation with the
doctor will be like. In the simplest terms, these consultations can be
described as the patient P consulting the doctor D about a problem of Ps. In
order for D to offer solutions to the problem, P must first describe it, and D
must ensure that he or she has enough information of an appropriate nature
to be able to categorise the problem, which then allows for a solution (or at
least a course of action or range of options) to be identified as appropriate
in the case of problems like Ps. The next stage in the process will involve D
communicating a possible solution (or range of solutions) to P and a nego-
tiation between P and D to arrive at a satisfactory outcome for both.

This is a very rough description of an ideal type of consultation. The
interest of discourse analysts lies in exploring the ways in which talk gets

---

Box 1.1 Standardised forms of notation

(.)   indicates a pause of less than two seconds; numerals in round brackets
      indicate the length of other pauses in seconds
[ ]   contains relevant contextual information or unclear phrases
[ ]   describes a non-verbal utterance
[between lines of dialogue indicates overlapping speech
<u>the</u>   underlining signifies emphasis
=   means that the phrase is contiguous with the preceding phrase without
      pause
:   indicates elongation of the preceding sound

things done (or not) in particular situations, thus it helps to outline the expectations that both participants bring to an encounter by virtue of being members of the same culture and sharing the same knowledge about how things get done; this knowledge is referred to by Fairclough (1992) as 'members' resources', following Garfinkel (1967).

The extract we examine is taken from a twelve-minute consultation, slightly longer than the average UK consultation duration which is somewhere between six and ten minutes. You will notice that it is characterised by short turns, many interruptions, and that neither speaker has long stretches of talk.

Female clinician (age 27) with female patient (age 52): 17 December 1999, twelve-minute duration

D: Doctor   P: Patient

[knock on door]
001 D: come in
002 P: hello
003 D: hello [door closes] (2.0) have you seen the lady outside
004 P: yes [yes]
005 D: [yes] you're happy about that
006 P: yeah
007 D: OK fine have a seat
008 P: [it's fine]
009 D: [good] (.) right ho- how are you
010 P: oh bit better
011 D: yeah how your husband doing
012 P: oh he's fine now [apparently (.) yes yeah no problems at all]
013 D: [is he he's comple<u>tel</u>y recovered (.) good so that]'s one stress [that's settled
014 P: [yeah ye:::s that's (.) yeah thank heavens] for that
015 D: down a bit (.) oh that's goo::d]
016 P: well a- <u>yes</u> he is (.hhh) but I'm y- know I'm sort of feeling a bit (1.0) I was
017   like that=
018 D: [right
019 P: (.hhh) but (1.0) <u>now</u> I I get very agitated (1.0) [just before a peri]od
020 D: [yes right (1.0)] abou- ho- how <u>lo::ng</u> before your period
021 P: uh:::- about a week
022 D: rig[ht]
023 P: [well uh <u>build</u>ing up to it so that <u>week</u> be[fore
024 D: [righ]t (.) an how soon does it disappear when the period starts

025 P: uhh about two days
026 D: OK=
027 P: =y- know I can feel it sort of (1.0) moving away [then]
028 D: [right] (.hhh) an so you say you're agitated you feel uptight
        are[you sleeping=
029 P: [well I'm (.) I'm absolutely terrible to live with I'm terrible to live
        with (1.0)]=
030 D: or (1.0) ri:::ght]
031 P: =I don't no:::rmally swear (.) but I (.) [you know I can get quite
        uh]
032 D: [(that's OK]
033 P: (.hhh)
034 D: so you find um I mean over the last few months the problem has
        seemed to have been
035 more consistent [hasn't it]=
036 P: [(emphatically) ye:::s::]
037 D: =[but you find]
038 P: [since I've been tak]ing the HRT
039 D: you've fou[nd that tha[t's a bit more of a problem]
040 P: [yes:: (1.0) yes::] because I've never suffered [from it ever in my life=
041 D: [right so (.) (that may be the cause)]
042 D: so when did you start the HRT then
043 P: oh gosh (.) oh I think it be nearly a year [now]=
044 D: =[right] so for this year [you've had (.) the symptoms]
045 P: [yeah (.) I- well this la::st three] (.) well t two months perhaps I-
        cos I was going to mention
046 it to you last time I saw you but everything (er) went wrong (.hhh)
        but er it's just this la::st sort
047 of three months I've [notic]ed=
048 D: [right]
049 P: t=hat just before (.) I could (.) [sort of kill somebody (1.0) sort of
        thing]=
050 D: [you feel (1.0) right OK right]
051 P: =but I've never suffered with it [before] so it really didn't occur to me=
052 D: =that that's what it wa[s
053 P: [no]
054 D: right (.) are your periods regular
055 P: yes
056 D: [they are (.) with the (.) H]RT
057 P: [yeah (.) yes yeah]=
058 D: =and are they any problem are they heavy or (.) t[roublesome any-
        thing (.)
059 P: [(emphatically) no:: bett::er cos I was losing a lot before but they
        (.) –re=

060 D: right that sounds a bit (refresh[ing) OK]
061 P: fine now (1.0) yeah yeah]
062 D: any bleeding bet<u>ween</u> the periods
063 P: no
064 D: little discharg[es or things like that [so=
065 P: [(coughs) excuse me (1.0) yeah fine yeah (1.0) yeah]
066 D: physically everything's works (1.0) fine it's just] those sort of
       symptoms that you're getting otherwise

To illustrate the process of analysing the discourse we will examine the opening sequence in detail (lines 1–8). Discourse analysis, drawing on insights from
conversation analysis, has recognised that talk is orderly and follows regular
patterns, known as the 'sequential organisation'. We will draw attention to the
relevant features of sequential organisation in our analysis. It has been found
that talk is both 'context shaped and context renewing' (Heritage 1984: 242),
a feature that allows speakers and hearers to coordinate their talk in a way
that makes sense to both. Hearers and speakers pay careful attention to each
utterance and *design* their turn to respond to the previous utterance and to
shape the next. For analysts this means that the meaning a hearer has given to
an utterance can only be determined by observing the next utterance or turn.
The fact that talk is organised in this coordinated fashion does not mean that
misunderstandings do not occur, but the analysis at least allows us to see just
how they occur and are 'repaired' (Schegloff *et al.* 1977; Schegloff 1992;
Edwards 1997). In summarising this, Edwards (1997) says:

> Within talk's publicly managed procedures, whatever meanings are
> taken up turn by turn by participants (for example in second speakers'
> turns) are also available for repair by first speakers in subsequent (for
> example, third) turns. Given the turn by turn possibility of repair its
> absence signals that participants are treating their talk as, by default,
> continuously coherent.
>
> (Edwards 1997: 101)

Conversely, we might expect that where many attempts at repair are recognisable we see that the conversation lacks continuous coherence and the
establishment of shared meaning between the participants is compromised.

As well as in repair, the sequential organisation of talk is also displayed
in 'adjacency pairs'. Adjacency pairs is the term to refer to turns where once
the first part of a pair is spoken, we normatively expect that a second part
will follow, for example a question creates the first part of a pair which is
completed by a response, as does an invitation to which the second part is
expected to be an acceptance or refusal (Sacks *et al.* 1974).

The sample sequence opens with the knock at the door that is the
patient's request for entry (first turn). The knock is taken as the first part

of a two-part sequence or 'adjacency pair' and we can anticipate that the next turn will be shaped by that original turn and will be a response to it. In our example, the doctor's response completes the pair – a knock requesting entry leads to a positive response. The next turn is initiated as the patient offers a verbal greeting and the doctor responds by returning the greeting. However, while this response would normatively be enough to have completed the turn and we might expect that the floor (or right to speak) would now be returned to the patient, after a two-second pause, during which the patient closes the door, the doctor extends her turn and asks a question. This means that the balance of right to speak first (and to set the agenda, for at least the next turn), has been taken by the doctor and that the patient's turn is now shaped by the need to respond to the doctor's request about whether she has 'seen the lady outside', who was ensuring that patients had been informed about the study. The patient confirms that she has indeed seen the researcher. The doctor moves to another question which is constructed as if to offer an answer to the patient that is already formulated as a positive response, by asking: 'you're happy about that'. This is a move that we describe in everyday talk as a rhetorical question, so-called because it is not really formulated as a question, but rather indicates a preferred answer. The phrase 'you're happy with that' signals to the patient the answer that is desired by the doctor. It would require significant interactional work on the behalf of the patient to refuse to comply with this stated assumption (see for example Goody 1978). This utterance of the doctor's is also characterised by a feature seen throughout the consultation, namely interruption. The doctor begins to speak before the patient has completed her utterance (notation symbols indicate overlap). It is a norm that one person speaks until their utterance is complete: interruption by a second speaker will mean that the first speaker will cease to speak. The technique is a powerful means of limiting speech (and in this case the opportunity to offer information) and is a feature that permeates the consultation.

We therefore see mechanisms that offer us insights into the way in which this consultation is being conducted. Many authors have pointed to the imbalance of power that exists between doctors and patients and the ways in which patients are disadvantaged; some have suggested that power is withheld from the patient by the doctor's failure to communicate effectively (Mishler 1984; Treichler et al. 1984; Heath 1992). Others have claimed that the imbalance of power is related to factors such as differences in gender and social class between patients and doctors, as well as differential knowledge. Some suggest that it is possible to shift the lack of equilibrium by employing techniques such as those described in the consultation process known as shared decision making (Elwyn et al. 1999). In the case of the transcript examined in this chapter, the doctor involved is attempting to use just such an approach but without any degree of success. It is in a case such as this that the very different perspective offered by discourse analysis can be extremely illuminating and helpful. It is unlikely that the doctor had thought about the impact of asking the question about consent before the patient had been invited to take her seat, and much less likely that the consequence of offering pre-formulated answers to questions had been pointed out to her by any form of feedback mechanism. The interruptions to the patient's turns also serve to work against a shared orientation to the consultation. As we can see, it is a frequently recurring feature of this consultation that the doctor offers answers to her own questions or completes the patient's turns for her, offering candidate or suggested responses of her own rather than allowing the patient the time to formulate her own responses, as for example in lines 39 and 52.

There are a number of possible reasons for this pattern, but the impact of talking in this way is to control the patient's turns in such a way that the patient never gets to tell her story without interruption, reshaping or reformulating by the doctor. It is important to emphasise that the features that discourse analysts are able to study are not intuitively available to speakers, but are the cumulative result of years of concentrated study. However, the opportunity now exists, building on this body of knowledge, to encourage practitioners to become aware of these features and for training that facilitates development of more productive patterns of talk.

The importance of narrative is another aspect of discourse analysis which is also being developed (Riessman 1993; van Langenhove and Harre 1993; Radley and Billig 1996; Edwards 1997). It offers useful insights for practitioners concerned to improve their communication skills. Narrative analysis directs our attention to how patients (and most people in interaction) prefer to describe their problem in a way that allows them to contextualise the technical description of symptoms in a storyline. To an extent, the work of the doctor in collecting information about a patient's problem can be compared with disembedding from the patient's account those pieces of information that can be linked to fit a medical framework, essentially a diagnosis or a problem formulation (Mishler 1984; Elwyn and Gwyn 1998). In the transcript, the patient makes several attempts to construct her account but is frequently thwarted as the doctor tries to gather data about symptoms without allowing her to finish. These interruptions could be seen as an attempt by the doctor to work more efficiently, but unless the patient is allowed time to formulate her own and specific experience, it is unlikely that a perception of jointly held understanding of problems presented will develop.

More examples of doctor control occur in lines 9–11 when the patient is asked 'How are you?' As the patient begins to answer, having marked the beginning of the turn with 'oh', which is a marker of dispreference, signalling that the answer is likely to be complicated in some way rather than a straightforward positive response, the doctor interrupts. This interruption changes the topic and leads to another question about the patient's husband. This removes the right to speak – what is termed the 'floor' – from the patient once again and also signals that the doctor is controlling the encounter rather than allowing the patient space and time to develop her story. At line 16, the patient attempts again to steer the consultation towards her concerns and she begins to describe her symptoms: this move can be termed 'repair' work. The patient is behaving as though the doctor's continued questions and changes of topic 'mean' that the patient has not sufficiently described her symptoms and concerns. She therefore makes a number of fresh attempts to convey the relevant information, which she feels will be needed to deal appropriately with her problem. This type of repair is identifiable throughout the consultation and should alert us to the possibility that the attempt by both participants to establish shared understandings of the consultation has been compromised.

Although we do not have the space to reproduce the full transcript, the patient's turns are frequently interrupted by the doctor, who completes the patient's sentences for her and repeatedly asks questions that cut short the patient's attempts to describe her symptoms and problem. At line 45 the patient attempts a slightly longer turn, and explains that on her previous visit 'I was going to mention it to you (...) but everything went wrong'. This would seem to offer any listener a clue to the fact that these consultations are flawed and that the patient is not being afforded the opportunity to achieve a satisfactory outcome, at least in terms of describing just what her problem is. Following this turn, the consultation returns once more to the pattern of very short turns as the doctor continues to ask questions which are related to the physiology of the woman's condition, allowing little scope for the development of her emotional and psychological concerns. The consultation, as we have already said, is longer than average, but there are no turns that extend beyond three lines; most of the longer turns are actually the doctor's. The longest patient turn without interruption is two lines. The consultation is fragmented, neither participant is afforded a long turn of talk (or listening). The outcome seems to be that the patient, who has repeatedly attempted to reveal more concerns, accepts the doctor's reformulation that she has 'premenstrual' symptoms and that altering her hormone replacement therapy may help.

In our second example the patient is a middle-aged woman and the consultation is shorter.

Extract from transcript of consultation (duration seven minutes)

D: Doctor   P: Patient

```
047 D:  I'm going to give you something called Augmentin
048     it's a little white bullet (.)
049     if you take them three times a day (.) [
050 P:  Mhm
051 D:  And we'll see if it helps you.
052 P:  OK that's lovely. [coughs briefly]
053 D:  Anything else?
054     (.)
055 P:  Uh (.) dya dya oh is it Dyazide (.)
056     the (.) water tablets I'm on?
057 D:  You take those regularly?
058 P:  Yeah every day (.)
059     now I always take them in the morning but (.)
060     would it be all right to take them in the night? (.)
061     you know because oh [sighing]
062     it drives me mad you know
063     'cause I (.)pass water so much=
064 D:  ='Course you do=
065 P:  =And as I say if I'm on holiday I think well
066     I don't want to be running into the toilet all the time.
067 D:  Why are you taking (.)water tablets?
068 P:  Because I'm on HRT?
069 D:  O yeah=
070 P:  =Um (.)clif clif cilafin is it? Well I've got enough of those. (.) [
071 D:  Mmm:mm.
072 P:  But I wanted the er Seroxat
073     the antidepressant tablets please.
074 D:  You take those do you?
075 P:  Yeah.
076 D:  How long have you been taking those?
077 P:  (.)Uh: well my son was killed (2.0) five years ago (2.0)
078     just after that then (.)three months after (.)
079     my (.)granddaughter
080     three month old twin granddaughter died of meningitis (.)
081     then in the January (.)my son in law got uh
082     died of a heart complaint
083     twenty two so I refused to take anything you know
084     but then (.)doctor Y insisted (.)
085     and I have found them and I started work
086     after thirty years I'm a receptionist at the um
```

087   [names famous Welsh institution] (.)
088   and I have <u>really</u> found that <u>that</u> has (.)
089   been <u>more</u> of a help to me (.)[breathes heavily]
090   but doctor Y said she <u>still</u> wanted me to take those antidepressants
091   but I was thinking (.)would I be able to take <u>one</u> one day
092   leave one off the next day
093   to try and (.)would you know
094   would that be all right do you think or?
095 D: Do you want to do that?

Even by examining this short extract the differences are clearly recognisable. There are much longer stretches of talk. Notice that the patient coughs briefly at the point where it may have been assumed that the business of the consultation was over and the doctor responds to this cough by offering the patient a further opportunity to take the floor by asking 'Anything else?' (line 53) (Elwyn and Gwyn 1998: 165–75). After a two-second pause (an unusually long pause in medical interactions), the patient begins a new topic by asking a question about medication; the doctor allows her to complete her query without interruption and responds with a clarification question. The patient goes on to request an antidepressant and the doctor asks her how long she has been taking this therapy, a question, like those of the doctor in the previous example, which is clearly oriented to time, but which the patient answers in terms of a narrative which contextualises her taking of the antidepressants firmly in terms of her life events (Gwyn 2002). The previous patient also attempted to respond to a question about time in line 20 ('How long before your period?') by beginning a narrative which allowed her to contextualise the technical question about time (temporal) in terms of her emotional state (lines 23, 29, 31). There is the possibility that, like our second patient, given the chance to describe the situation in her own terms she might have also suggested a possible solution or at least given voice to the crux of her problems. The first patient, however, is cut short by the series of questions that the doctor uses to refine the temporal timing of the problem, thus overriding the patient's attempt to describe subjective issues that are pertinent to her. In our second extract the patient is allowed to describe her problem without interruption. This allows a narrative to emerge which is packed with information which, although it may not necessarily correspond with a diagnostic framework, clearly offers the doctor a wealth of information which allows him to understand the request to reduce antidepressant medication. Acting on this information he is able to offer the patient support for the decision that she is suggesting.

The analysis of these two extracts has considered a very restricted sample of features from discourse analysis in order to enhance our common-sense understanding of these two consultations. We have looked at the overall time taken by the consultations, which speaker spoke most often and for how long, turn taking, interruptions, questions, repair and the ways in which patients seek to narrate their experience. We therefore propose that discourse analysis offers a valuable counterbalance to approaches that deal with fragments or segments of a communication event. Not only does discourse analysis recognise the need to treat interactions as meaningful constructs within specific contexts, but it is also able to explore the mechanisms in interaction itself and the way in which turns are designed and influenced by the subtle signals employed by speakers. Understanding is part of the way to changing, and this is where we turn next.

Implications and new directions

These two extracts provide insight into communication strategies employed by the healthcare professionals that lie beyond a quantitative analysis. The analysis illuminates the way the practitioners interact with patients, revealing how in one example the opportunities for drawing out the essential narrative are lost, whilst in the other the patient is allowed not only a space in which to describe her predicament, but is also facilitated to explore and examine the meaning of her narrative. The use of discourse analysis as an academic means to research institutional talk and communication strategies has been extremely important. It has, nevertheless, typically remained closed off from the practitioner world. Examining transcripts in great detail, with findings reported in journals and conferences, is outside the orbits of the practitioners themselves. They are largely unaware of the discipline of discourse analysis, its aim, and more importantly the impact it could have on professional practices if dialogue could be created between analysis and practitioners.

There are, however, developments taking place at the more practical end, where the techniques of discourse analysis are used in training settings, although the techniques as a necessity are significantly modified. Box 1.2 describes the use of these techniques within a communication skills unit in a general practice teaching unit and Box 1.3 lists the features of the training.

Given the enormous influence of communication on the effectiveness of the delivery of healthcare it is clear that focused efforts such as those described above are worth exploring and evaluating. Whilst a body of academic work exists in which researchers explore health professionals' use of language in a variety of contexts and its impact on both colleagues and patients (Silverman 1987; Griffiths 1997; Griffiths 1998; Griffiths 2001), relatively little has been carried out in collaboration with health professionals with a view to improving their own practice. The work of Rollnick and others described above explores these techniques in relation to general practice, but we believe the techniques and approaches described in this chapter are also highly relevant for any health or social care, or indeed human service work context.

Box 1.2 Context-bound training

The term context-bound training describes the integration of two concepts. First, practitioners are encouraged to train in their own contexts (workplaces) so that they generate scenarios and problems that are as specific and relevant as possible to their day-to-day settings. They are encouraged to specify the communication issues that they want to address, thereby doing their own real-time needs assessment. At this stage, simulated patients are asked to work with the practitioners to construct scenarios that are the basis of simulated consultations. These consultations are conducted at the training session and are then transcribed, typically overnight, so that the transcripts are available for review on the following day. By using detailed transcripts, the trainers and the practitioners review the communication strategies and reflect on where the practitioner has done well and where there is room for modification or improvement. Video could be used in a similar way but the impact of video is more overwhelming and immediate, and the medium does not allow time to reflect on turn-taking strategies, interruption and back-channelling techniques (all the 'ums' and 'ahs' in conversation). The use of these transcripts, albeit rudimentary in terms of detail compared to academic analytical texts, allows both practitioners and trainers to reflect and learn more about individual communication skills and how to modify them (Rollnick *et al.* 2002a; Rollnick *et al.* 2002b).

Box 1.3 Features of context-bound training

• Participants work in same/similar environment	Essential
• Participants willing to see actor alone before and after group discussion	Essential
• Practitioners agree to listen to recording or read transcript before meeting with colleagues and trainer(s)	Essential
• Participants willing to discuss experiences with colleagues and trainer(s) in group meeting	Essential
• Feasible to collect recordings of simulated consultations	Essential
• Trainer able and willing to integrate own material with experiences of participants in simulated consultations	Essential
• Actors able to visit practitioners on-site	Highly desirable
• Participants willing to provide scenario(s) beforehand	Highly desirable
• Group discussion meeting held on-site	Desirable
• Trainer able to listen to recordings or read transcripts beforehand (in confidence)	Desirable
• Actors able to provide feedback (recorded, in person or in writing)	Optional
• Trainer available to discuss progress and experiences on individual basis	Optional

Jones (2003) has explored the ways in which conversation analysis can be utilised by nurses to reflect on their own communicative practice in admitting patients to hospital, and students are able to benefit from opportunities to analyse anonymised transcripts, but it is entirely possible that short courses in communication skills, such as those described above, could be included in all human service work training. There is also a case to be made for incorporating such training into continuing professional development. Most medical schools have realised the need to invest energy and expertise in communication skills units. There are, therefore, parallel challenges for other healthcare professionals. We communicate with exquisite skill and execute our aims efficiently, often without realising the power differentials and the impact of our interruptions and back-channelling efforts. The skills of listening, of developing means to allow patients to deliver their explanatory narratives, do not necessarily come from watching videotapes. These communication strategies are best studied at a pace that allows individuals to examine their turns and pauses in more depth. We contend that you do not need to read many transcripts to know your weaknesses. Discourse analysis, suitably modified, can be a tool for improving healthcare communication.

References

Boon, H. and Stewart, M. (1998) 'Patient–physician communication assessment instruments: 1986 to 1996 in review', *Patient Education and Counseling*, 35: 161–76.

Byrne, P. S. and Long, B. E. L. (1976) *Doctors Talking to Patients*, London: Her Majesty's Stationery Office.

Drew, P. and Heritage, J., eds (1992) *Talk at Work: Interaction in Institutional Settings. Studies in Interactional Sociolinguistics*, no. 8. Cambridge: Cambridge University Press.

Edwards, D. (1997) *Discourse and Cognition*, London: Sage Publications.

Elwyn, G. and Gwyn, R. (1998) 'Stories we hear and stories we tell ...', in Greenhalgh, T. and Hurwitz, B., eds, *Narrative Based Medicine*, London: BMJ Publications.

Elwyn, G., Edwards, A. and Kinnersley, P. (1999) 'Shared decision making: The neglected second half of the consultation', *British Journal of General Practice*, 49: 477–82.

Fairclough, N. (1992) *Discourse and Social Change*, Cambridge: Polity Press.

Garfinkel, H. (1967) *Studies in Ethnomethodology*, Englewood Cliffs, NJ: Prentice Hall.

Goody, E. N., ed. (1978) *Questions and Politeness: Strategies in Social Interaction*, Cambridge: Cambridge University Press.

Griffiths, L. (1997) 'Accomplishing team: Teamwork and categorisation in two community mental health teams', *The Sociological Review*, 45: 59–78.

Griffiths, L. (1998) 'Humour as resistance to professional dominance in community mental health teams', *Sociology of Health & Illness*, 20: 874–95.

Griffiths, L. (2001) 'Categorising to exclude: The discursive construction of cases in community mental health teams', *Sociology of Health and Illness*, 23: 678–700.

Gwyn, R. (2002) *Communicating Health and Illness*, London: Sage Publications.

Harre, R. and Stearns, P. (1995) *Discursive Psychology in Practice*, London: Sage Publications.

Heath, C. (1992) 'The delivery and reception of diagnosis in the general practice consultation', in Drew, P. and Heritage, J., eds, *Talk at Work: Interaction in Institutional Settings. Studies in Interactional Sociolinguistics*, no. 8, Cambridge: Cambridge University Press.

Heritage, J. C. (1984) *Garfinkel and Ethnomethodology*, Cambridge: Polity Press.

Inui, T. S. and Carter, W. B. (1985) 'Problems and prospects for health service research on provider–patient communication', *Medical Care*, 23: 521–38.

Jones, A. (2003) 'Nurses talking to patients: Exploring conversation analysis as a means of researching nurse–patient communication', *International Journal of Nursing Studies* (forthcoming).

Kurtz, S., Silverman, J. and Draper, J. (1998) *Teaching and Learning Communication Skills in Medicine*, Abingdon, Oxon: Radcliffe Medical Press.

Mishler, E. (1984) *The Discourse of Medicine: Dialectics of Medical Interviews*, Norwood, NJ: Ablex.

Nessa, J. and Malterud, K. (1990) 'Discourse analysis in general practice: A socio-linguistic approach', *Family Practice*, 7: 77–83.

Potter, J. (1996) *Representing Reality*, London: Sage Publications.

Radley, A. and Billig, M. (1996) 'Accounts of health and illness: Dilemmas and representations', *Sociology of Health and Illness*, 18: 220–40.

Riessman, C. K. (1993) *Narrative Analysis*, London: Sage Publications.

Rollnick, S., Kinnersley, P. and Butler, C. C. (2002a) 'Context-bound communication skills training: Development of a new method', *Medical Education*, 9, 36: 377–83.

Rollnick, S., Seale, C., Kinnersley, P., Rees, M., Butler, C., and Hood, K. (2002b) 'Developing a new line of patter: Can doctors change their consultations for sore throat?', *Medical Education*, July, 36, 7: 678–81.

Roter, D. L. (1991) *The Roter Method of Interaction Process Analysis*, Baltimore: John Hopkins University, Department of Health Policy and Management.

Sacks, H. (1989) 'Harvey Sacks: Lectures 1964–65', in Jefferson, G., ed., *Human Studies*, 12, 3–4 (special issue): 183–404.

Sacks, H. (1992) *Lectures on Conversation*, Oxford: Blackwell.

Sacks, H., Schegloff, E. A. and Jefferson, G. (1974) 'A simplest systematics for the organisation of turn-taking in conversation', *Language*, 50: 697–735.

Schegloff, E. A. (1992) 'Repair after next turn: The last structurally provided defence of intersubjectivity in conversation', *American Journal of Sociology*, 97: 1295–345.

Schegloff, E. A., Jefferson, G. and Sacks, H. (1977) 'The preference for self-correction in the organisation of repair in conversation', *Language*, 53: 361–82.

Silverman, D. (1987) *Communication and Medical Practice: Social Relations and the Clinic*, Bristol: Sage Publications.

Stewart, M., Brown, J. B., Weston, W. W., McWinney, I. R., McWilliam, C. L. and Freeman, T. R. (1995) *Patient Centred Medicine: Transforming the Clinical Method*, Thousand Oaks, CA: Sage Publications.

Treichler, P., Frankel, R., Kramarae, C., Koppi, K. and Beckman, H. (1984) 'Problem and problems: Power relationships in a medical encounter', in Kramarae, C., Schulz, M. and O'Barr, W. M., eds, *Language and Power*, London: Sage Publications.

van Langenhove, L. and Harre, R. (1993) 'Positioning and autobiography: Telling your life', in Coupland, N. and Nussbaum, J. F., eds, *Discourse and Lifespan Identity*, London: Sage Publications.

Waitzkin, H. (1990) 'On studying the discourse of medical encounters. A critique of quantitative and qualitative methods and a proposal for reasonable compromise', *Medical Care*, 28: 473–88.

Wooffitt, R. (1992) *Telling Tales of the Unexpected*, Hertfordshire: Harvester Wheatsheaf.

Chapter 2

The turn to a narrative knowing of persons

Minimalist passive interviewing technique and team analysis of narrative qualitative data[1]

Kip Jones

> A person does not ... stand motionless and clear before our eyes with his
> merits, his defects, his plans, his intentions with regard to ourself
> exposed on his surface ... but is a shadow which we can never succeed in
> penetrating ... a shadow behind which we can alternately imagine, with
> equal justification, that there burns the flame of hatred and of love.
>
> (Marcel Proust, *The Guermantes Way, Part I* (1920))

According to Denzin (2001: 23), the turn to narrative in the social sciences
has been taken, is a fait accompli. One result of this paradigm shift is a
renewed interest in biography as a method of knowing persons. Denzin
(2001: 30) points out that 'no longer does the writer-as-interviewer hide
behind the question–answer format [or the semi-structured probe], the apparatuses of the interview machine'. Finally, therefore, the interviewer has
become a willing participant in a dialogic process. Narrative biography or
'storytelling' offers up the opportunity for democratising the experience of
teller and listener (or performer and audience) by sharing the goal of participating in an experience, which reveals shared 'same-ness' (Porter cited in
Denzin 2001: 25). This has been expressed by Scheff (1997: 219) as the concept of the '*habitus* – our second nature, the mass of conventions, beliefs and
attitudes which each member of a society shares with every other member'.
The paradox thus develops that by expressing individual differences we
uncover common ground.

The use of biographical methods to promote participatory and inclusive
approaches to health and social care research has been hailed as ground-
breaking, particularly in documenting hidden histories and dialogue with
disparate communities (Rickard 2002: 2). Chamberlayne and King (2000: 9)
comment that 'the rising popularity of biographical research tools may well
lie in their aptness for exploring subjective and cultural formations, and tracing interconnections between the personal and the social'. It is the view of

Miller (2000: xii) too, that using a biographical approach to understanding human concerns makes sense in that its methodology transcends the barriers of self/society as well as those of past/present/future. These include 'barriers between the individual self and the collective society as well as those compartmentalising the past, present and future' (Miller 2000: xii). In addition, Jones (2001a: 1) notes that the grounding of narrative studies in theoretical and philosophical principles has persisted in flourishing since the early 1990s.

There is a danger, however, in the assumption that 'business as usual' approaches to qualitative enquiries need simply tack the word 'narrative' to titles of qualitative studies to result in them becoming narrative enquiries. The gold standard of 'semi-structured probes' used in much social science interview research in the past several decades, is too often based upon the predetermined assumptions built into the researcher's questions (cf. Priest 2000: 245), one of Denzin's 'apparatuses of the interview machine'. The turn to narrative enquiry shifts the very presence of the researcher from knowledge-privileged investigator to a reflective position of passive participant/audience member in the storytelling process. The interviewer as writer/storyteller then emerges later in the process through her/his retelling of the story as a weaver of tales, a collage-maker or a narrator of the narrations.

The interview/case-study approach selected for the author's PhD research, 'Narratives of identity and the informal care role' (Jones 2001b), is based on training in a method of biographical narrative interviewing and analysis developed by Chamberlayne and Wengraf at the Centre for Biography in Social Policy, University of East London – the biographic narrative interpretive method (Chamberlayne *et al.* 2000; Wengraf 2001). This method, in turn, is built upon a method developed in Germany in the early 1990s by Rosenthal and others, which evolved from Shuetze's 1976 method of story and text analysis and Oevermann's 1980 objective hermeneutical case reconstruction (Rosenthal and Bar-On 1992: 109). It is a dynamic and interpretive method, with an emphasis on action and latent meaning, which distinguishes it within the broad and rich range of life history, oral history and narrative approaches (Chamberlayne and King 2000: 17). According to Miller, this:

> objective hermeneutic method proceeds on a step-by-step basis, with each supposition or proto-hypothesis being immediately evaluated against interview transcript material – 'hermeneutic' since the researcher is aware that any material being produced by the interviewee has been generated with regard to both the interviewee's subjective perception of her/his situation and history and the interviewee's perception of the research and the relationship between the two of them.
>
> (Miller 2000: 131)

I chose this particular narrative interview method for my research because it incorporated the possibility of working with two key concepts: first, that stories are unique and individually constructed wholes, and second, that what interviewees have to say about their lives and self-concepts is much more illuminating than any specific research assumptions or questions could be. For example, I may have had preconceived ideas or questions about what an interviewee's life as a carer might be. The carer her/himself may, on the other hand, have seen the constructed whole of her/his life story as one as, for example, a parent, daughter, son and so forth, not just the story of her/his carer role. This role, in fact, may well have been one constructed or nested within another more central role or one left undefined and separate from it.

Overview of the biographic narrative interpretive method

Interview technique in the biographic narrative interpretive method uses a single, initial, narrative-inducing, 'minimalist-passive' question (Wengraf 2001: 113), for example, '*Tell me the story of your life,*' to illicit an extensive, uninterrupted narration. Miller comments that:

> This apparently simple request has led to a quiet revolution in social science practice. For it even to be seen as a legitimate query required a shift in paradigmatic viewpoints about the nature of the social scientific enterprise.
>
> Miller (2000: 1)

A technique of non-interruption then maintains the 'gestalt' of the participant's story. Gestalt has been defined by Hollway and Jefferson (2000: 34) as 'a whole which is more than the sum of its parts, an order or hidden agenda informing each person's life', and is central to the theoretical principles of the biographic narrative interpretive method. Gestalt represents the constructed shape of a story, through theme, motif and/or various agendas – hidden or otherwise. In the biographic narrative interpretive method, the first part of the interview is followed by a second sub-session, based upon the gestalt of the first and reflecting the ordering of themes presented by the interviewee in the initial interview. After the second interview sub-session, additional material can then be used to build the case, including the possibility of a follow-up third session with more focused probes as well as the collection and discussion of ancillary materials such as diaries, writings and photographs.

In the view of Murray and Holmes:

> Eliciting open-ended narratives provides a window on the very structure of individuals' representations ... stories allow researchers to see the gestalt – the interrelations of structural linkages that individuals perceive among positive and negative attributes and experiences.
>
> Murray and Holmes (1994: 660)

This very shift encompasses willingness on the part of the researcher to cede 'control' of the interview scene to the interviewee and assume the posture of active listener/audience participant. This claim not to probe, guide or ask questions and its potential for revealing the flux and contradictions of everyday subjective reality, is in itself a theoretical orientation closely allied to symbolic interactionism (Plummer 1983: 123).

Microanalysis of the narrative of the reconstructed life follows the interview stage, using a reflective team approach to data analysis. The 'lived life', or chronological chain of events as narrated, is analysed sequentially and separately. The 'told story', or thematic ordering of the narration, is then analysed using thematic field analysis, involving reconstructing the participants' system of knowledge, their interpretations of their lives and their classification of experiences into thematic fields (Rosenthal 1993: 61). Rosenthal defines the thematic field as: 'the sum of events or situations presented in connection with the themes that form the background or horizon against which the theme stands out as the central focus' (1993: 64).

Miller describes how narrative biography has evolved from concepts of life history and life story:

> Originally, life *story* referred to the account given by an individual about his or her life. When this personal account was backed up by additional external sources ... the validated life story was called a life *history*. This concern with triangulation – the validation of narrated life stories through information from additional, preferably quantified, sources has not remained central to most current biographical practice. Nowadays ... 'life history' refers to a series of substantive events arranged in chronological order ... 'Life story' still refers to the account given by an individual, only with emphasis upon the ordering into themes or topics that the individual chooses to adopt or omit as s/he tells the story.
>
> Miller (2000: 19)

Rosenthal (1993: 61) points out that 'life story and life history always come together. They are continuously dialectically linked and produce each other; this is the reason why we must reconstruct both levels no matter whether our main target is the life history or the life story.' The biographical details and themes are tested against in-depth analysis of the text, examining hesitancy, repetition, contradictions and pauses. Through hypothesising how the lived life informs the told story, the case history is then finally constructed from the two separate threads of the 'lived life' and the 'told story'. A case structure is then formulated that validates more than one event based upon the actions of the interviewee.

Other narrative approaches

Mishler (1995: 87) exclaims, 'this is an exciting time for narrative researchers, a period of rapid growth in the number and variety of narrative studies in the human sciences.' He describes a typology of approaches to narrative studies that focuses on which of three alternative problems are defined as the central task for narrative research:

- reference and the relation between temporal ordering of events and their narrative representation;
- textual coherence and structure, and how these are achieved through narrative strategies;
- psychological, cultural and social contexts and functions of narratives.

Within each of these general categories, subclasses are distinguished in terms of the specific ways in which the central problem is addressed (Mishler 1995: 87).

An in-depth recounting of Mishler's typologies will not be attempted here, except to say that within the subclass of *psychological, cultural and social contexts*, the category *narrativisation of experience: cognition, memory, self* paralleled the aims of my informal care research. Key to this category is 'the construction of a personal narrative as central to the development of one's self, of an identity' (Mishler 1995: 108) and this resonated with my project's goals. Additionally, Mishler states that reports of this process typically take the form of summaries of 'cases' (1995: 109).

Miller (2000) proposes another typology of the approaches to biographical investigation: *realist, neo-positivist* and *narrative* approaches. The realist approach uses unfocused interviews, focused around grounded theory techniques, and is, therefore, inductive; the neo-positive approach uses focused interviews, is deductive and theory-testing; and the narrative approach emphasises the active construction of life stories through the interplay of interviewer and interviewee where the past and future are seen through the lens of the present (Miller 2000: 10–13). As Miller asserts, 'the three approaches delineated above can overlap considerably in practice' (2000: 14), however, there are real differences of substance between them (2000: 18).

The approach chosen for my informal care research (the biographic narrative interpretive method) has resonance with Miller's narrative approach. Although distance is maintained between the interviewer and interviewee by the nature of the single-probe/active-listening interview, the interplay between the interviewer and interviewee is still a central concern, albeit not until analysis. This minimal approach still acknowledges that the interviewer's characteristics are bound to affect the course of the interview and that this should be recognised (Miller 2000: 101). Rosenthal (cited in Miller 2000: 129) supports this with the assertion that 'ultimately each interview is a product of the mutual interaction between speaker and listener'.

McAdams (1996) has devised a framework for the narrative study of persons that includes investigating the psychosocial construction of life stories by means of which modern adults create identity. McAdams (McAdams *et al.* 1997: 679) proposes that personality description encompasses at least three independent levels: (a) dispositional traits, such as the Big Five;[2] (b) contextualised concerns, such as developmental tasks and personal strivings; and (c) integrative narratives of the self. The third level (narrative) is the level of identity. McAdams (1996), in analysing more than 200 accounts from life-story interviews, proposes the following as structural features of the content of life stories: narrative tone, imagery, themes, ideological setting, nuclear episodes, images and endings (1996: 308–9). McAdams *et al.* (1997) have also developed a conceptual model of generativity, based in Erikson's stage theory, as a constellation of seven psychosocial features, centred round the personal and societal goal of providing for the next generation (1997: 680).

McAdams *et al.* (1997) combine qualitative emphases with the conventions of quantitative research by use of quantitative content analysis of the narrative data, and include the convention of a control group (1997: 681). The narrative-gathering process itself asks the participant to divide her/his life into 'chapters', provide a title and plot summary for each, and delineate and describe eight specific scenes or nuclear episodes within the divisions of high point and low point, turning point, earliest memory, and significant childhood, adolescent, adult and other memories. Next, the participant is asked to identify and describe the four people who have had the biggest impact on her/his story and to identify a personal heroine or hero. After that, the participant is asked to describe what she/he sees as the future chapters of the story. The process continues, asking for more specific stories related to such areas as hopes, dreams, areas of conflict, ideology, religious beliefs, political views and philosophy, and finally, a possible dominant theme or message in the whole of the story.

McAdams seeks a 'methodological and epistemological middle ground' and believes that 'careful' research can lead to the kinds of interpretations that are useful for life stories (1997: 690). Although I find the methodological underpinnings in McAdams' work to be consistent with the aims of my own work, I found the method itself to be less useful.

Hermans *et al.* (1992) conceive the self as a dialogical narrator constructed by a multiplicity of dialogically interacting selves with the other not outside but in the self-structure, resulting in the multiplicity of selves (1992: 23). Hermans (2000: 4) describes three suppositions that underlie his narrative approach:

- Stories acknowledge both the perception of reality and the power of imagination.
- Space and time are basic components of storytelling.

- Both the storyteller and the actors in the stories are intentional beings who are motivated to reach particular goals which function as organising story themes in their narratives.

Hermans nests a narrative theory of the self, based on the metaphor of the motivated storyteller, in his valuation theory. 'The notion of story is expressed in the central term "valuation" as a process of meaning construction' (2000: 8). Hermans uses a self-confrontation method in which a person is invited to perform a thorough self-investigation by constructing a set of valuations, elicited by a series of open-ended questions, rating each of the valuations and discussing the results (2000: 8–9). Hermans' (Hermans and Kempen 1993: 149) self-confrontation method, like McAdams' method, is based on a combination of qualitative data (valuations) and quantitative data (affective indices). Hermans states that his valuation theory is not a final theory: 'it is devised as an open framework in development ... to investigate a diversity of psychological phenomena as a process of organization, disorganization, or reorganization of the valuation system' (1993: 23). Hermans' research takes place in a clinical setting and is therefore more therapeutically constructed than was the design of my informal care research.

Hollway and Jefferson (2000) base their narrative work in the theories of psychoanalyst Melanie Klein about how the self is forged out of unconscious defences against anxiety – the 'defended subject' (2000: 19). These defences are intersubjective, that is, they come into play in relations between people (2000: 20). The authors incorporate Klein's concept of the defended subject within their narrative method. Based loosely upon Chamberlayne and Wengraf's biographic narrative interpretive method, Hollway and Jefferson's narrative method makes a case for the relationship between people's ambiguous representations and their experiences or 'critical realism' (2000: 3). The inner and outer worlds of their subjects make up what the authors term the 'psychosocial' (2000: 4).

Hollway and Jefferson make use of free associations in order to elicit hidden meanings and incorporate the defended subject within the biographical narrative interpretative method. Thus, ultimately, the authors remain indebted to psychoanalysis, both theoretically and methodologically. Their 'subjects' are not only positioned within the surrounding social discourses, but are also seen as motivated by unconscious investments and defences against anxiety. The data production is based upon the principle of free association, and data analysis is dependent upon interpretation (2000: 77).

Hollway and Jefferson champion methodological tools that parallel psychoanalysis, including the unconscious, intersubjective dynamics of the interview relationship and therapeutic concepts such as counter transference, recognition and containment. The authors make a case for using 'a method based on the principle of working with the whole data and paying attention to links and contradictions with that whole' (2000: 5), in contrast to the widespread tendency in qualitative research to fragment data by using code and retrieve methods which use software programmes to look for patterns and identify themes in textual data obtained from interviews, observations, surveys, journals and other documents in order to aid researchers in analysing textual data.

The work of Hollway and Jefferson is important to my research in that it solidifies concepts of reflective practice within the narrative interviewing experience and clearly delineates psychoanalytical concepts useful to a social psychological approach to interpretation in narrative biography. In addition, these authors' successful reinterpretation of and expansion upon the original Chamberlayne and Wengraf method is helpful in substantiating my project's diversions from the originating method.

Sample size

Because the biographic narrative interpretive method requires extensive interviews with follow-up sessions, as well as intricate and labour-intensive analytical procedures, sample frames typically remain small. Often a sample size is projected initially, but remains fluid throughout the research process (Benner 1994: 107). Factors affecting the ultimate number of cases presented include the size of the text that was generated, the number of colleagues involved and their availability. For analysis to be thorough and meaningful, these colleagues must be assembled into reflecting teams to explore and hypothesise themes. This, combined with the richness of data presented, often necessitates the limiting of the number of interviews to be analysed in full. Efforts can be made, nonetheless, to insure that the initial selection of subjects for interview includes a diverse range of participants with varying demographic and family relationship backgrounds (Chamberlayne and King 2000: 16–17). For the purpose of my research, seven informal carers of widely different cultural backgrounds, ages and familial roles were interviewed. What may have been lost in not using a method with the potential for handling larger numbers of subjects, so producing large data sets, was more than compensated by the method's capacity for generating deep and meaningful case studies. These are rich with potential for the discovery of new material and for the generation of further hypotheses, for effecting change in social policy and ultimately validating and illuminating participants' lives.

Interviewing

The interview procedure in my research, based upon the biographic narrative interpretive method, began with the single probe:

I would like you to tell me the story of your life. Take as much time as you would like. I am not going to interrupt you, but I will be taking notes. When you are finished, we will take a break for about 15–20 minutes. When we resume, I will be asking you a few more details based upon my notes of what you have told me.

As interviewer, I made no further interjections except for confirming utterances, making eye contact and unconscious body language. If a participant was 'stuck' and did not know what to say or how to go on, phrases such as 'take your time' were used to reassure the participant, but no new questions were posed. Such attentive listening 'draws the stories out of their hide-away … expectant listening seems to be an indigenous part of all stories or narratives' (Wyatt in Sarbin 1986: 200). Crucially, the gestalt of the participant's story was maintained by this method of non-interruption. By balancing and linking these two central concepts of minimalist–passive interviewing (maintenance of the gestalt of the storyteller and drawing her/him out through expectant listening), a revolution in interview technique is accomplished.

For my research, most initial interview sessions lasted between 45 and 60 minutes. Usually, the session ended by the participant stating, 'that's about it', or 'well, that's my story'. In all cases it was the interviewee who ended the session. Silences were maintained without interjection by the interviewer, unless the participant asked for help. In these instances, phrases such as 'well, tell me more about your life' were used to help the participant. Mishler (in Sarbin 1986: 235) makes the point that 'if we allow respondents to continue in their own way until they indicate they have finished their answer, we are likely to find stories; if we cut them off … if we do not appear to be listening to their stories … then we are unlikely to find stories.'

Between the first and second sessions, participants were asked to fill out a single-sided questionnaire of background information. During this time, the interviewer read through the notes taken in session one and looked for developing themes and phrases or areas of story that could be expanded upon. After the break, the participant reattached the microphone and the second part of the session began. The themes and stories to be elaborated upon were presented in the same order, using the same words that the participant had used in sub-session one, and therefore maintaining the gestalt of the narrative established in the earlier session. Typically, the second part of the interview lasted 30–45 minutes. The session ended with the interviewer asking if there was anything that the participant would like to add or felt that s/he had missed. If there was not, the interviewer then suggested that a follow-up telephone call could be made in case any further input from the participant was desired and to have an opportunity to correct any biographical details such as names and dates. The participant was then thanked and the session ended. At a later date, a thank-you letter was sent to the participant and the promised follow-up phone call was made.

In certain circumstances, when important underdeveloped themes of a particular interview suggest productive follow-up questions, a third interview session is necessary. Wengraf (2001: 204) elaborates: 'Although the three sub-sessions are analytically distinct from the point of view of the researcher–interviewer, they do not necessarily mean that the interviewee will experience all or only three apparently different interviews. Typically, sub-sessions one and two blend together into a "first interview" and sub-session three is a "second interview"'. At this second interview (or third sub-session), it is possible to probe for more specific information that takes into account the 'read' of the initial sessions and the interviewer's impressions of the lived life and told story. Because this is the first time that the interviewer's responses to the manifested data form questions, the gestalt of the told story is not interrupted or broken.

In one of the author's early cases, a follow-up third sub-session was held to test the method to its widest extent, but also to expand upon and enrich the material from the earlier two sessions. It was at this time and place that, finally, I directly responded to the participant's story with enquiries based on my reflections and early interpretations. The questions were based on dialogue from the story as presented in the original sessions, although not necessarily in the same order. Themes were drawn together and presented as probes, encouraging the participant to relate to the possible connections indicated by the interviewer's questions – based upon early interpretations of several possible themes. In this particular case, the participant was asked to bring photographs and documents to the third session for discussion, exploration and elaboration of the life story. As Mishler indicates, such ancillary materials 'acquired outside the boundary of the interview but still within the boundaries of the study' (Mishler cited by Sarbin 1986: 247) are crucial in building a case. In this instance, photographs were particularly helpful in unearthing periods or stories in the participant's past that had been difficult to convey during the first sessions.

Post-interview processes

I compiled session debriefing notes as soon after each session as possible in order to get down on paper the initial feelings, responses, concerns and so forth raised by the interview. I listened to the recorded interview and took notes from the second hearing. When I typed the word-for-word transcript, I also made notes. These initial debriefings are necessary and central to understanding the interview process, providing an opportunity for the interviewer to express ideas about the session, including obstructions (Wengraf 2000: 39). The accumulated notes became crucial documents for later reflection by me and supported the use of relational metaphors in understanding 'the problem', the actions taken (or not) and the relationships 'among the interlocutors themselves' (Gergen 1999: 8).

Next, the biographical data chronology of the life story was compiled. It was here that a biography (names, dates, events and so forth) was constructed in chronological order and in a brief note format. Finally, the text structure sequentialisation of the story was constructed – a diagram 'showing the changing structure of the text, particularly that of the story told in the initial narration' (Wengraf 2001: 236). This is a textural structure created freely by the interviewee and reflects the gestalt of the told story. It includes, but is not limited to, changes in speaker, topic change and/or 'text sort' change, or change in the way a given topic is being treated by the speaker through *description*, *argumentation*, *report*, *narrative* or *evaluation* (Wengraf 2001: 241).

During and immediately following the period of the University of East London training, I conducted an exploratory full pilot interview (a three sub-session interview process that took place on two separate days). Because of the complicated medical history of the participant's husband, questions arose concerning her version of his medical story. It was decided to set up a 'case study' session based upon the participant's narrative description of her husband's illness. Two medical doctors in a general practice research group at the university were asked to participate in a pilot analysis/reflecting team session. The session was conducted in order to familiarise me with the process, to test the method's applicability to the data at hand and as a means of being able to begin to help me understand the health history of the interviewee's husband.

Initial reservations about the flexibility of the medical doctors to participate in a pointedly qualitative process were dissipated by their immediate grasp of the analytical process and method's concept. In fact, Hunter (in Mishler 1995: 112–13) has reminded us that medicine is made up of stories and is dependent on narrative – essentially case-based knowledge and practice – and that clinical judgement is 'fundamentally interpretative' (1995: 112–13). An hour-long session based upon eight to ten lines of transcript provided a means of achieving rich hypothesising as well as generating materials for further analyses. Benner (1994: xviii) suggested that 'once an interpretation of a text is developed, one may engage in a comparison of that interpretation with any other level of theoretical or cultural discourse offering critical reflection and comparison with the interpretive commentary'.

Data analysis

Glaser and Strauss's often invoked grounded theory derives from analytic induction (Chalip in White *et al.* 1998: 3) and analytic induction is also the basis of the data analysis method used in the biographic narrative interpretive method. Analytic induction was first described by the sociologist Florian Znaniecki in 1934 (Ratcliff 2001: 1; Robinson 1951: 812). The analysing of human documents (letters, memoirs, life histories) was used extensively by Znaniecki in the second decade of the twentieth century in his seminal work, *The Polish Peasant in Europe and America* (Thomas and Znaniecki 1958 [originally published 1918–20]). This approach to life and lived experience was later defined as the autobiographical method in sociology and located in the theory of symbolic interactionism (Plummer 1983: 40). Znaniecki was a faculty member of the University of Chicago at the time when its department of sociology – the first of its kind in the United States – was known as 'the Chicago School'. The life history method was central to this department (Miller 2000: 4), which was the first in an American university to establish an original, collective school of thought: pragmatism (Plummer 1983: 51). Znaniecki's approach stimulated debate within both sociology and psychology for several decades. For example, the psychologist Allport advocated, more strongly than anybody else, the use of idiographic (dealing with the individual) case study method in psychology. He proposed that its use overcame the pursuit of general laws about traits abstracted from individuals, which had ignored the unique constellation of traits in one individual (Plummer 1983: 48). Znaniecki held the view that analytic induction is the true method of the physical and biological sciences, and that it ought to be the method of the social sciences too (Znaniecki cited in Robinson 1951: 812). Inductive rather than deductive reasoning is involved, allowing for modification of concepts and relationships between concepts. The process occurs throughout the action of doing research, with the goal of most accurately representing the reality of the situation. No analysis is considered final, since reality is constantly changing. The emphasis in analytic induction is on *the whole*, even though elements and the relationships between elements are analysed. A specific case need not necessarily be representative of the general phenomena studied. It is crucial, nonetheless, that a case has essential characteristics and that it functions as a pattern by which future cases can be defined (Robinson 1951: 1).

Znaniecki's analytic induction process was seen by Cressey in 1950 as comprising six steps (cf. Ratcliff 2001: 1):

1   A phenomenon is defined in a tentative manner.
2   A hypothesis is developed about it.
3   A single instance is considered to determine if the hypothesis is confirmed.
4   If the hypothesis fails to be confirmed, either the phenomenon is redefined or the hypothesis is revised to include the instance examined.
5   Additional cases are examined and, if the new hypothesis is repeatedly confirmed, some degree of certainty about the hypothesis results.
6   Each negative case requires that the hypothesis be reformulated until there are no exceptions.

Chamberlayne (Chamberlayne and Rustin 1999: 25) makes the claim that the biographic narrative interpretive method is based, in part, on grounded theory. I found, however, that returning to its basis in analytic induction was more productive in my own work. In fact, analytic induction is different from the now more widely used grounded theory (Glaser and Strauss 1967) in several ways. Analytic induction tests, as well as generates, theory and all data available must be used to test hypotheses (Ratcliff 2001: 2). Furthermore, 'in interpretive (hermeneutic) research, unlike in grounded theory, the goal is to discover meaning and to achieve understanding' (Benner 1994: 10). On the other hand, grounded theorists themselves may very well lay claim to goals of discovering meaning and achieving understanding.

Inductive data analysis, as an alternative to grounded theory's 'constant comparison method' (Thomas in White *et al.* 1998: 1) 'is typically qualitative; it makes use of comparisons (typically of cases); it often makes use of techniques which share some affinity with phenomenology and hermeneutics' (Chalip in White *et al.* 1998: 3). By using analytical induction within a phenomenological or hermeneutic approach, a philosophical statement is made about the underpinnings of the analysis (White in White *et al.* 1998: 5). It is, nonetheless, 'perfectly feasible to interpret data obtained via particular methods ... that are dissimilar from those who advocate (or even invented) those methods' (Chalip in White *et al.* 1998: 6). In addition, Becker (1958: 654) has shown that several ways of doing analysis in a study can be triangulated and this data used to speculate about what might be (1958: 654).

Analogous to Znaniecki's and Robinson's analytic induction technique, as well as the biographic narrative interpretive method, is Mehan's (cited in Ratcliff) 'constitutive ethnography' which incorporates aspects of analytic induction.

> The process of analysis is initiated with analysis of a small data set from which a tentative hypothetical framework is generated. Comparisons are made with additional forthcoming data resulting in changes in the framework until a group of 'recursive rules' are developed that comprehensively describe the phenomenon.
>
> (Ratcliff 2001: 2)

Reflecting teams

Using a 'reflecting team' approach to data analysis facilitates the introduction of multiple voices, unsettling and creating a mix of meaning and encouraging communication and collective means of deliberation (Gergen 2000: 4). In my research, reflecting teams, put in place in order to facilitate the group analytical process, were comprised of other researchers and faculty members solicited by me. The recruiting process begins by gathering colleagues (two, three or more per team) from varying professional and demographic backgrounds and immersing the teams in the transcript, at times line by line, hypothesising at each new revelation of dialogic material. What is sought through this procedure is an opening up of the possibilities in interpretation, rather than sole reliance upon the primary researcher's interpretation of an interview. The abilities required of group participants are openness and creativity/imagination rather than knowledge of specific research methods. In fact, diversity of approach to the material should be solicited and encouraged. In this way, each participant brings his or her own social context or 'lived life' to the process and, therefore, contributes uniquely to the ways of seeing the lives of others.

In my research, reflecting teams were solicited through the email lists of a research centre and the faculty of the university. The final group consisted of a pool of 19 people. Dates and times for sessions were established and coordinated with the schedules of interested respondents. The sessions, which took place over one year, lasted approximately three hours and were held at a campus location. Thirteen reflecting team meetings were held and four of the seven interviewee's transcripts were analysed. The lived life and told story were analysed in separate sessions using different reflecting teams.

The sessions began by introducing the participants, whose details were noted on a flip chart. Most teams comprised nurses, researchers and lecturers. The panel members were then asked to tell something about themselves that one might not expect from the earlier professional descriptions offered. These were also written on the flip chart. Participants were then asked to bring to the analysis session that 'other' person whom they had just described. Through this introductory exercise, they were encouraged to engage in a dialogue with the text of the life of another and bring to that dialogue more than just their professional selves. Some examples of the team participants' descriptions of their past experiences included the following: time spent as a surveyor; working as a male fashion model; immigrating from Zimbabwe; having spent childhood as an evangelical missionary; having formerly been a fine artist; having failed at A-levels; being raised as a Romany gypsy; and membership of a hippy commune. Some of these experiences were quite surprising, considering the team members' present activities and occupations. Participants ranged in age from those in their 20s to those in their 50s, with one participant nearing 70. Gender was equally represented in most sessions. Four participants were non-white.

An important and interesting lesson was learned from the reflective team sessions. If time ran out and the end of the transcript had not been reached, participants seemed somewhat dissatisfied. It became clear that team members needed to know the whole story – the beginning, middle and end – as in any good story. Another observation was that once team members were immersed in the process, their personalities came to the fore. For example, one member, who has a great sense of humour, often used humour or casual remarks when going through the exercise of hypothesising and analysing the transcript sentence by sentence. These seemingly flippant remarks often held a great deal of truth, unknown to the panel at that particular stage of data analysis. In addition, the oldest panel member seemed to impart a special wisdom to the process from the strength of his life experience, something others did not have in such abundance. It was also observed that some members with nursing backgrounds initially had difficulty projecting possible outcomes from early data in the lived life or told story. When questioned about this informally, they replied that their training made it difficult for them to make value judgements about the lives of others. Wengraf (in Chamberlayne *et al.* 2000: 144) comments on this type of situation thus:

> The value of the panel of analysts and of peer review lies, in part, in the capacity of different researchers to have anxieties that are different from those of each other and from that of the interviewee.
>
> (Chamberlayne *et al.* 2000: 144)

After some time working with the method, however, those with nursing backgrounds were able to find their own way of hypothesising.

In the process of using the biographic narrative interpretive method, individual and unique approaches to data analysis emerged. It became clear to me that certain aspects of the method often got in the way of the data's potential to inform and illuminate. Pragmatic considerations of working within a team setting produced a need to be flexible. In fact, the method's claim that it is an 'advance on the intuitive approach of much qualitative research in Britain' (Chamberlayne and King 2000: 10) raised further questions: in asking reflecting team members to speculate about a life story, was not the potential of intuition ultimately a great advantage to this very process (Scheff 1997: 33–6)?

The rigidity of Chamberlayne and Wengraf's text structure sequentialisation tool (Wengraf 2001: 239–43) made it unwieldy when producing data that was workable for the reflecting teams within the time allotted for analysis. The method seemed to require an adherence to consistencies within the told narrative, rather than uncovering links based on spontaneous association (Hollway and Jefferson 2000: 152). Concentrating on the text structure appeared to restrict the reflecting teams' possibilities of multiple, intuitive responses to the data. In addition, the configuration of the text structure sequentialisation seemed to be changing and becoming more complex with each new publication by its authors (Chamberlayne *et al.* 2000; Chamberlayne and King 2000; Wengraf 2000; Wengraf 2001). A decision was made, therefore, to reduce strict adherence to this particular process of the biographic narrative interpretive method and concentrate on the more instinctive and creative possibilities of the data analysis interface through selection of meaningful text upon which hypotheses and associations might be made – that is, using microanalysis.

For these pragmatic reasons, therefore, the text sequentialisation process was 'back grounded' and the microanalysis of selected text was 'fore grounded' within the team setting. According to Rupp and Jones (in Chamberlayne *et al.* 2000: 288), 'microanalysis aims at analysing the inter-relation between past experiences and their presentation in depth, concentrating on small selected pieces of text and checking previous hypotheses'. This process of abduction, or posing all possible hypotheses after each unit of text and then gradually eliminating them, necessitates the limiting of the microanalysis to small, selected extracts of text.

In certain instances during my research, the text chosen for analysis was selected because it did represent shifts in the modes of narration by the interviewee (description, narration, argumentation (Wengraf 2001: 239–43)). At other times, however, text was selected for its ability to telegraph potential themes and their development, or emotional states such as anxiety and defence (cf. Hollway and Jefferson 2000). In one case, for example, the interviewee's use of sighs and/or laughter was microanalysed for meaning and theme development by analysing the dialogue surrounding these physical utterances (cf. Jones 2001a). Nonetheless, all narrative microanalyses followed the order in which they were expressed by the interviewee.

Key to my particular investigation of personality and its commitment to the concept of the *individual within a social context* is the claim that all interpretive work, however sociological, requires a theory of the subject (Hollway and Jefferson 2000: 59). The centrality of the individual within a social context was imperative in illuminating my original research questions. In my subsequent inquiry, therefore, strict adherence to what in the end was a sociologically developed method seemed counterproductive to my study's social psychological agenda.

Conclusions

What does it mean when we know a person (Jones 2000)? In truth-seeking, are we merely comparing and contrasting our own everyday world with the worlds of others? Within the individual's world and her/his tendency of 'revealing/concealing', 'knowing/not knowing' (Heidegger in Krell 1993), by exploring the terrain, are we simply only portraying the process itself, its dialectical underpinnings, its thesis and antithesis? Or, in fact, do we, in our attempts at some sort of a truth (verismo), stumble on a synthesis after all, a moment of revelation that truly is wrenched by the individual in her/his self-knowing and revealed to us?

Asking a person to tell us about her/his life is just a beginning. By doing this, in a less than perfect way, we are at least starting by participating in the story of the person in her/his world, her/his expectations, successes, failures and dreams. The swirl of a remembered past is (re)constructed by just such illusive characteristics. A narration of a life is, when all is said, a story, an illusion. Freeman reminds us:

> Any and all stories we might tell *about* ourselves are essentially ficti-
> tious; they are vehicles for warding off the flux and meeting our need
> for order – illusory though it may be to suppose that this order exists
> anywhere but in our own minds.
>
> Freeman (1997: 379)

Veracity, therefore, must remain secondary. What remains primary is that this is how one individual sees her/himself when asked to recount her/him-self today (Plummer 1983: 57). Freeman (1993: 30) maintains: 'reflecting on one's life is fundamentally a metaphorical [process], giving form to one's previous and present experience'. As much as we try to elevate this metaphor to a discussion of objects, concepts, thoughts and the like, to a higher plane perhaps, by exploring meaning within meanings of the lan-guage used to describe such things, we all still 'bump into the furniture' (1993: 13). Perhaps the most any approach to knowing of others can pro-duce in sensing the lives of others – that very 'otherness' – is a fleeting consciousness of what it is like to bump into their furniture, their own 'selves' through the stories that they construct via the illusory imagination of narrative. These are the illusions like the shapes, forms and monsters that one envisions in passing clouds. They reform back into clouds again, and then pass from view, as we remain always expectant of another to appear. *'It's cloud illusions I recall'* (Mitchell 1969). The trick is to 'get it down', this illusion, this configuration of momentary meaningfulness, before it escapes from memory. Such it is in illusion: so too in life stories.

Freeman sums up thus:

> the project at hand is therefore ultimately a reconstructive one; it is a
> project of exploring lives in their various modes of integration and dis-
> integration, formation and de-formation, and, on the basis of what is
> observed, piecing together images of the whole.
>
> Freeman (1997: 395)

This whole becomes the imaginative subjective drama of an everyday life: the verismo of the quotidian. In listening to stories, like an anticipating audience ushered into the hush of a darkened theatre, our disbelief is mutu-ally suspended and the possibility of shared comprehension is embraced.

Notes

1 This chapter expands upon an earlier published journal article, 'The turn to a narrative knowing of persons: one method explored', *Nursing Times Research* (2003) 8, 1: 60–71. The author wishes to express his gratitude to Professor Robert Miller, Director of the Centre for Social Research, Queen's University, Belfast, for his helpful suggestions in reviewing the article.
2 The Big Five include: Extraversion/Surgency; Agreeableness; Conscientiousness; Emotional Stability; Intellect/Openness.
McAdams is known for his criticism of the Big Five dispositional traits as 'the psychology of the stranger'.

References

Becker, H. S. (1958) 'Problems of inference and proof in participant observation', *American Sociological Review,* 23: 652–60.
Benner, P., ed., (1994) *Interpretive Phenomenology: Embodiment, Caring, and Ethics in Health and Illness*, Thousand Oaks, London, New Delhi: Sage Publications.
Chamberlayne, P., Bornat, J. and Wengraf, T., eds (2000) *The Turn to Biographical Methods in Social Science: Comparative Issues and Examples*, New York: Routledge.
Chamberlayne, P. and King, A. (2000) *Cultures of Care: Biographies of Carers in Britain and the Two Germanies*, Bristol: Policy Press.
Chamberlayne, P. and Rustin, M. (1999) *From Biography to Social Policy*, Final report of the Social Strategies in Risk Society (SOSTRIS) project (SOE2-CT96-3010), University of East London, Centre for Biography in Social Policy.
Denzin, N. K. (2001) 'The reflexive interview and a performative social science', *Qualitative Research,* 1: 23–46.
Freeman, M. (1993) *Rewriting the Self History, Memory, Narrative*, London, New York: Routledge.
Freeman, M. (1997) 'Death, narrative integrity, and the radical challenge of self-understanding: A reading of Tolstoy's *Death of Ivan Illich*', *Ageing and Society,* 17: 373–98.
Gergen, K. J. (1999) 'Social construction and the transformation of identity politics', draft copy for Newman, F. and Holzman, L., eds, *End of Knowing: A New Developmental Way of Learning*, New York: Routledge. Available at: http://www.swarthmore.edu/SocSci/kgergen1/web/printer-friendly.phtml?id=manu8
Gergen, K. J. (2000) 'The poetic dimension: Therapeutic potentials', draft for Deissler, K. and McNamee, S., eds, *Phil und Sophie auf der Couch, Die soziale Poesie Therapeutischer Gesprache*. Heidelberg: Carl-Auer. Available at: http://www.swarthmore.edu/SocSci/kgergen1/web/printer-friendly.phtml?id=manu19.
Glaser, B. G. and Strauss, A. L. (1967) *The Discovery of Grounded Theory*, New York: Aldine.
Hermans, H. J. M. (2000) 'The person as a motivated storyteller: Valuation theory and the self-confrontation method', draft copy accessed (2000) at: http://www.socsci.kun.nl/hermans/Polyphony.html. Ch in Neimeyer, R. A. and Neimeyer, G. J., eds, *Advances in Personal Construct Psychology*, 2002 (pp. 3–38), Westport CT: Praeger Publishers.

Hermans, H. J. M. and Kempen, H. J. G. (1993) *The Dialogical Self Meaning as Movement*, San Diego, London: Academic Press.

Hermans, H. J. M., Kempen, H. J. G. and van Loon, R. J. P. (1992) 'The dialogical self beyond individualism and rationalism', *American Psychologist* 47, 1: 23–33.

Hollway, W. and Jefferson, T. (2000) *Doing Qualitative Research Differently: Free Association, Narrative and the Interview Method*, London: Sage Publications.

Jones, K. (2000) 'Big science or the bride stripped bare by her bachelors, even', review essay, *Forum: Qualitative Social Research* 1:3. Available at: http://www.qualitative-research.net/fqs-texte/3-00/3-00review-jones-e.htm.

Jones, K. (2001a) 'Beyond the text: An Artaudian take on the non-verbal clues revealed within the biographical interpretive process', paper presented at the International Sociological Association conference on methodological problems of biographical research, Kassel, Germany, 25 May. Available at: http://www.angelfire.com/zine/kipworld/Beyond_the_Text.htm.

Jones, K. (2001b) 'Narratives of identity and the informal care role', unpublished PhD Thesis, De Montfort University, Leicester.

Krell, D. F. (1993) *Basic Writings: Martin Heidegger*, London: Routledge.

McAdams, D. P. (1996) 'Personality, modernity, and the storied self: A contemporary framework for studying persons', *Psychological Inquiry*, 7, 4: 295–321.

McAdams, D. P., Diamond, A., de St. Aubin, E and Mansfield, E. (1997) 'Stories of commitment: The psychological construction of generative lives', *Journal of Personality and Social Psychology*, 72, 3: 678–94.

Miller, R. (2000) *Researching Life Stories and Family Histories*, London: Sage Publications.

Mishler, E. G. (1995) 'Models of narrative analysis: A typology', *Journal of Narrative and Life History*, 5, 2: 87–123.

Mitchell, J. (1969) 'Clouds', Siquomb Publishing Corp.

Murray, S. L. and Holmes, J. G. (1994) 'Storytelling in close relationships: The construction of confidence', *Personality and Social Psychology Bulletin*, 20: 650–63.

Plummer, K. (1983) *Documents of Life: An Introduction to the Problems and Literature of a Humanistic Method*, London: George Allen and Unwin.

Priest, H. M. (2001) 'The use of narrative in the study of caring: A critique', *Nursing Times Research*, 5, 4: 245–50.

Ratcliff, D. E. (2001) 'Analytic induction as a qualitative research method of analysis'. Available at: http://don.ratcliff.net/qual/analytic.html.

Rickard, W. (2002) 'The biographical turn in health studies', in draft for Ch. in P. Chamberlayne, J. Bornat and U. Apitzsch (eds), *Biographical Methods and Professional Practice*, forthcoming March 2004, New York and London: Routledge.

Robinson, W. S. (1951) 'The logical structure of analytic induction', *American Sociological Review*, 16: 12–18.

Rosenthal, G. (1993) 'Reconstruction of life stories: Principles of selection in generating stories for narrative biographical interviews', in Josselson, R. and Lieblich, A., eds, *The Narrative Study of Lives*, London: Sage Publications.

Rosenthal, G. and Bar-On, D. (1992) 'A biographical case study of a victimizer's daughter's strategy: Pseudo-identification with the victims of the Holocaust', *Journal of Narrative and Life History*, 2, 2: 105–27.

Sarbin, T. R. (1986) *Narrative Psychology: The Storied Nature of Human Conduct*, New York, Westport, London: Praeger Publishers.

Scheff, T. J. (1997) *Emotions, the Social Bond, and Human Reality: Part/Whole Analysis*, Cambridge: Cambridge University Press.

Thomas, W. I. and Znaniecki, F. (1958) *The Polish Peasant in Europe and America*, New York: Dover Publications (first published 1918–20).

Wengraf, T. (2000) 'Short guide to biographical-narrative interviewing and analysis by the SQUAIN-BIM method', unpublished training manual, University of East London: Centre for Biography in Social Policy.

Wengraf, T. (2001) *Qualitative Research Interviewing Biographic Narrative and Semi-Structured Methods*, London: Sage Publications.

White, G., Chalip, L. and Marshall, S. (1998) 'Grounded theory and qualitative data analysis', electronic discussion. Health Research Methods Advising Service (HRMAS) Newsletters (Numbers 9, 10, 11), August. Accessed 2000 at: http://www.auckland.ac.nz/mch/hrmas/qual2d.htm.

Chapter 3

Hermeneutics and nursing research

Hugh Chadderton

The past 15 years have seen increasing numbers of nurses using hermeneutics as the philosophical foundations for their research. Since the pioneering work by Benner (1985), 25 Heideggerian studies were published between 1987 and 1997 in journals indexed in the Cumulative Index for Nursing and Allied Health Literature (CINAHL) (Drauker 1999) and then a further 19 Heideggerian and Gadamerian studies added to that figure between 1998 and 2003. The use of hermeneutics appears to be largely associated with nurses undertaking doctoral education, though a few studies are associated with Master's level study. As well as long courses, Professor Nancy Diekelmann has, since 1990, offered yearly short courses in Heideggerian and Gadamerian hermeneutics at the University of Wisconsin-Madison. The beginning (basic) course lasts 10 working days and attracts 15–20 international students; the advanced course lasts five days and attracts 35–40 international students. Many doctoral students attend the beginning course to get a sense of direction for their studies and then return to the advanced course to consider new calls to thinking.

This chapter now traces the history of hermeneutics before reviewing a sample of studies where the researchers stated they used hermeneutics to underpin their work. The chapter is in five sections. The first section considers the ancient origins of hermeneutics in the activities of the messenger-god Hermes and the priests at Delphi; it also deconstructs the term interpretation. The second section considers the periods of biblical exegesis. The third section reviews the work of Freidrich Schleiermacher, who made textual interpretation the concern of philosophy. The fourth section considers modern hermeneutics through the projects of Edmund Husserl, Martin Heidegger and Hans-Georg Gadamer. The fifth section is a review of 14 research studies conducted by nurses about phenomena of interest to nursing. Readers should note that the history of hermeneutics is limited to work in the Greek, German and English-speaking worlds and for the periods stated.

Ancient origins of hermeneutics

There are two sources of the word hermeneutics in Greek myths and legends. The first source is the word *hermios*, which refers to priests at the Oracle at Delphi to whom the Greeks went for advice. The second source is the word *hermeneia*, which relates to the messenger-god Hermes who interpreted the messages of the gods for mortals, lead the dead to the River Styx and guided travellers on their journeys (Palmer 2002). Hermes was the illegitimate son of Zeus and the nymph Maia and is often depicted as an athletic young man dressed in a winged hat and winged sandals (Grant and Hazel 1994). Hermes had not, however, always been cast in the role of messenger-god, as this was performed by the rainbow-goddess Iris. He was given the job by Zeus to keep him out of trouble after exploits such as stealing Apollo's cattle and sacrificing them. But he is probably best known in the role of messenger, guide and interpreter.

In considering the term 'interpretation', Palmer (1969) argued that this is a modern and heavily compressed term to signify saying, explaining and translating. In respect of the saying component, Palmer suggested that the term *herme* is etymologically close to *sermo* (to say), which reflects the oral tradition of the ancient Greeks and the bringing-of-the-word by Hermes and the priests at Delphi. Grondin (1995) developed this theme, arguing that the oral tradition leads to the idea of a reader bringing expression to text just as a musician interprets a piece of music, whether it is played from the stave or memory. In respect of the explaining component, Palmer argued that in the act of interpretation, a reader will often draw on the understanding of those present to illustrate an argument and that this happens in writing too, when the writer draws on previous conversations or previously read texts. In illustrating this argument he used the example of the teaching of Jesus, who, when speaking about Old Testament writers and his hopes for the salvation of humankind, would draw on the hopes of listeners in his audience to illustrate his points. Concerning the translation component of interpretation, Grondin (1995) reasoned that because Greek culture was homogeneous, the ancient Greeks showed little interest in languages other than their own and translation should not be considered in the modern-day context as the translation of other languages. She added that *translatio* was in fact a Roman word to signify a movement across the latitudes, specifically, movement across the Adriatic Sea. What did interest the ancient Greeks however, was the thought that language had meaning that travelled beyond the individual spoken or written word.

Periods of biblical exegesis

Palmer (1969) called the next two periods in the development of hermeneutics, from the death of Christ to circa AD700 and then on to the late Middle

Ages, the periods of biblical exegesis. Reader (1988) briefly considered the first period, stating that the schools of biblical interpretation ranged against each other at this time. McGrath (1997) elaborated, explaining that the Alexandrian school founded by the Greek-speaking Jewish philosopher Philo of Alexandria (30BC to AD45) was established in the belief that God uses religious scholars to communicate His word. This led to the school supplementing literal interpretation of the Bible with allegorical interpretation, making God's word meaningful in context and therefore accessible to a larger audience. The Antiochene school on the other hand, founded by Lucien (AD240 to 312), was developed in the belief that Christ used only a literal interpretation of the older texts and that the allegorical school needed to be held in check. The school promoted literal interpretations of the Bible that made no concessions to context.

In the second period, from AD700 to the Middle Ages, the allegorical school developed a method for interpretation known as the Quadriga or fourfold sense of Scripture. This addressed the literal sense of the Bible, its allegorical meaning, its moral meaning and an anagogical or uplifting meaning that gave Christians hopeful messages about what they could expect from life (McGrath 1997). These developments in the religious world attracted the attention of secular academics, who gradually began to draw on methods of biblical exegesis for the interpretation of classical texts, creating what Palmer (1969) described as 'classical' philology. Classical philology was initially used only with complex texts but later became a method for the interpretation of any text.

Freidrich Schleiermacher

Freidrich Schleiermacher was born in Breslau in 1768. He read theology at the University of Halle in 1790 before becoming a private tutor and curate. He moved to the University of Würzburg in 1804 to become professor, before moving again to Berlin where he was influential in establishing the university. He was appointed professor there in 1810, a role which he combined with that of pastor at the Trinity Church. He died in Berlin in 1834.

Schleiermacher's contribution to hermeneutics was made up of three parts. The first part was his appreciation that hermeneutics is more than just textual interpretation. Kimmerle (1977) noted that he was probably the first person to express the view that hermeneutics is primarily about the conditions of understanding, thereby making it the concern of philosophy. The second part was his belief that hermeneutics had the potential to be a general method that could be used to understand any text. This point was made in his address to the Prussian Academy of Sciences in 1829:

> Hermeneutics does not apply exclusively to classical studies, nor is it merely a part of this restricted philological organon; rather it is to be

applied to the works of every author. ... We can come to learn a great deal from works which have no outstanding intellectual content, for example, from stories narrated in a style similar to that normally used in ordinary conversation to tell about minor occurrences ... or [from] letters composed in a highly intimate and casual style.

(Schleiermacher [1833] 1977: 181)

Schleiermacher was later criticised for this approach, for whilst on the one hand he was attempting to broaden the uses of hermeneutics, on the other he was also concerned to develop universal laws of interpretation. The development of such laws was seen to run counter to the priority given to the historical circumstances of the text and the reader (Palmer 1969). The third part of his contribution was the appreciation that all understanding involves considering both the part and the whole. In his compendium of teaching notes of 1819, Schleiermacher made what is probably the first reference to the hermeneutic circle:

1 Complete knowledge always involves an apparent circle, that each part can be understood only out of the whole to which it belongs, and vice versa. All knowledge which is scientific must be constructed in this way.
2 To put oneself in the position of an author means to follow through with this relationship between the whole and the parts. Thus it follows, first, that the more we learn about an author, the better equipped we are for interpretation, but second, that a text can never be understood right away. On the contrary, every reading puts us in a better position to understand because it increases our knowledge.

(Schleiermacher [1833] 1977: 113)

There are three issues associated with Schleiermacher's approach to text that are relevant to nursing research. The first is that it is not only written text that can be interpreted, but anything made. This is illustrated by Diamond (1992) and Gubrium (1997) who each, as part of larger studies, considered the layout of nursing homes and how it affected the people who lived and worked there, and by Highley and Ferentz (1988) and Nelson (1996) who used photo-hermeneutics as an approach to enquiry. The second issue is that mis-understanding of text is the rule and that it is unlikely that any text will be understood on first reading. The need for reading and re-reading is empha-sised by Burnard (1991), whilst Diekelmann, Allen and Tanner (1989) and Gullickson (1993) not only recommended reading and re-reading, but also that interview transcripts should be read aloud. The third issue concerns the relationship of text to context, for Schleiermacher argued that ideas in a text should be considered in the context in which they occur and that the study of parallel texts will enable the interpreter to understand better the author and his or her relationships. In his study of the Being of older people in nursing homes, Chadderton (2003) examined narratives from older people, relatives and nurses in the context of the relevant gerontology, social geography and phenomenology literature. This led him to new literature on space, place and dwelling, which he then used to interpret the narratives.

Modern hermeneutics

The development of modern hermeneutics is most closely associated with the projects of Martin Heidegger, Hans-Georg Gadamer and those who have critically assessed their work. It may seem rather odd then, to include the work of a philosopher whose ideas at first appear to be at variance with hermeneutical thinking. There are two reasons for including the work of Edmund Husserl in this history of hermeneutics. The first is to clarify what is meant by Husserlian phenomenology, as this term is sometimes used interchangeably with Heideggerian phenomenology and Gadamerian hermeneutics (Koch 1995). The second is to consider what Grondin (1995: 35) describes as Husserl's 'silent contribution' to hermeneutics and the relevance of his work in modern hermeneutical thinking.

Edmund Husserl

Edmund Husserl was born in Prosnitz in 1859. Having studied astronomy and mathematics at the universities of Leipzig, Berlin and Vienna (Sandmyer 1998), he then studied psychology before being appointed full professor at the University of Göttingen. Alston and Nakhnikian (1964) speculate that Husserl's career had stalled in the first years of the new century and that it was in Göttingen that he determined to make a lasting contribution to philosophy. Husserl moved to the University of Freiburg in 1916. He retired in 1928 and died in 1938.

Alston and Nakhnikian (1964) argued that Husserl's phenomenology, first described in five lectures at the University of Göttingen in 1907, could be seen as an attack on psychology. They argued that Husserl believed that the discipline of psychology was attempting to reduce the laws of logic to generalisations about the way people think and feel and that nothing should be inferred without rules of inference. Husserl's own view, however, was that the starting point for his phenomenology was Cartesian subjectivism:

> Without doubt there is a *cogitatio*, there is namely a mental process during the subject's undergoing it and in a simple reflection upon it. The seeing, direct grasping and having of the *cogitatio* is already a cognition. The *cogitationes* are the first data.
>
> (Husserl [1907] 1964: 2)

Husserl argued that the seeing *cogitatio* expresses a real immanence, whilst everyday experiences and the sciences overlay or blur this seeing with theories of their own, in a process called transcendence. From that point on, his project was concerned not with the empirical nature of things, or the transcendence created by those who theorise, but with investigating the bare data of cognition and how these could be accessed. By the time of his inaugural address at the University of Freiburg in 1917, Husserl had sufficiently developed his project to be able to state:

> It would be the task of phenomenology, therefore, to investigate how something perceived, something remembered, something phantasied, something pictorially represented ... looks as such, i.e. to investigate how it looks by virtue of that bestowal of sense and of characteristics which is carried out intrinsically by the perceiving, the remembering, the phantasying, the pictorial representing etc. of itself.
>
> (Husserl [1907] 1964: 3)

Concerning how to reach the self-givenness of phenomena, Husserl ([1907] 1964) described a series of steps that he believed left immanence bare to see. The first step was to suspend belief and disbelief about the phenomenon in question. This *bracketing-out* served to exclude the transcendencies imposed by everyday understanding and the elaborate theories developed by the natural and human sciences. The second step was a device called *eidetic reduction*, whereby the phenomenologist attempted to determine the essential elements of a phenomenon by imagining it to take various forms that are manipulated until the form ceases to exemplify the phenomenon. Paley (1997) noted that this step is also called 'free variation', whilst Streubert and Carpenter (1995) used the term 'imaginative variation' for the same manoeuvre. The third step involved a final act of phenomenological reduction, where, freed from transcendencies and clear about form, the phenomenologist was able to make valid assertions about the self-givenness or essence of the phenomenon in question.

Problems with Husserlian phenomenology

There are, however, two problems with the Husserlian phenomenology. The first is that it is solipsistic (Paley 1997). This means that any explanation of things in the phenomenologist's world is dependent on the consciousness of the phenomenologist alone. The second (Alston and Nakhnikian 1964: xxii) is that it was naive of Husserl to assume that objects, feelings and other phenomena exist independently of the language that describes them and that language should not be seen as an instrument or something that 'the phenomenologist can create at will in the image of the ultimate facts'. These problems notwithstanding, Husserlian phenomenology has been advocated as a suitable approach for guiding nursing research (Omery 1983; Swanson-Kauffman and Schonwald 1988; Rose, Beeby and Parker 1995) and has been cited as the theoretical framework used in several nursing research studies including those of anorexia (Santopino 1988), community health nursing (Streubert 1991) and comfort (Morse, Borttoff and Hutchinson 1994).

Koch (1995) voiced concern about the way in which some nurse researchers approached Husserlian phenomenology, saying they tended to describe it in terms of methods and techniques of analysis developed from psychology rather than by the philosophical assumptions underpinning the methods. As a result, she added, not only were the foundations left unexplored, but the differences between Husserlian and other phenomenologies were left unexplored as well. Paley (1997) extended this criticism by claiming that on the basis of an examination of the published research, many nurse researchers appeared to misunderstand the concepts underpinning Husserlian phenomenology and although Husserl's authority was often invoked, usually in terms of bracketing, his work was rarely referenced directly. As a result, Paley claimed, many Husserlian research studies 'come close to being unintelligible'.

Turning to what Grondin (1995) called Husserl's *silent* contribution to the development of hermeneutics, it is difficult to see how a solipsistic theory with so little regard for language could make any contribution to the development of understanding. But at the heart of Husserlian phenomenology there is the challenge to 'detach oneself from the deforming hold of theories' (Grondin 1995: 35) and in so doing, move away from superimposed interpretations to see what is essential in the phenomena in question. Expressed another way, there is, in the call to strip off the layers of transcendence to the immanence below, an appreciation that understanding is a part of Being and that it is Being that provides the key to understanding. This is the contribution that Husserl made to the development of hermeneutics.

Martin Heidegger

Martin Heidegger was born in Messkirch in 1889. He went to the University of Freiburg to read theology but changed to major in philosophy, receiving his doctorate in 1913 (Krell 1996). In 1922 he accepted an associate professorship at the University of Marburg. On publication of *Being and Time* in 1927 he was awarded a full professorship. Declining a chair at the University of Berlin in 1930 he accepted the rectorship of the University of Freiburg, a post which he held for less than one year (Sheehan 1988). He remained at the university until 1945. He died at his home in Freiburg in 1976.

The challenge to Husserl and the formulation of 'Dasein'

During the time as his assistant, Heidegger began to question Husserl's phenomenology. There were two reasons for this. The first was that Husserl's teaching had become stylised, with practical classes in phenomenological seeing taking the place of philosophical debate. The second was that Heidegger knew that the ancient Greeks had conceptualised understanding quite differently, with phenomena becoming manifest through a process of *aletheia* or unconcealedness. Heidegger continued to question the grounding of phenomenology over the next few years and by the time he had become an associate professor at the University of Marburg, he had 'achieved three decisive insights' (Krell 1996: 17).

The first insight was that Husserl was not wrong to assert the importance of going back to the things themselves, but that the *logos* of phenomenology was not Cartesian subjectivism but the way phenomena make themselves manifest through unconcealment. Palmer (1969: 128) expressed this clearly when he said that it was not a case of the mind projecting meaning onto a phenomenon, rather what appears is the 'ontological manifesting of the thing itself'. Moreover, it was through language that phenomena come out of concealment into the light of day. The second insight was that truth in phenomenology was not a matter of the correctness of assertions at the end of a phenomenological reduction, nor any kind of agreement between subject and object, but the fact that phenomena had become unconcealed in the first place. The third insight was however the most radical, with Heidegger arguing that as phenomenology unconceals what *is*, at this *time* and in so doing, it answers questions of Being. Krell explained Heidegger's conception of Being this way:

> Heidegger resisted the traditional ways of talking about the Being of man in Christian dogma, Cartesian subjectivism, or the disciplines of anthropology and psychology, in order to concentrate on man's character as the questioner. Man questions his own Being and that of other things in the world. He is always, in no matter how vague a way, aware of his being in the world. Heidegger called the Being in general of this questioner ... *Dasein*.
>
> (Krell 1996: 19)

Before considering the role of language in the unconcealing of Being and asking what relevance this has to hermeneutics, it is important to understand what Heidegger meant by Being and how this relates to the German word *Dasein*. To understand Heidegger's conception of Being it is necessary to go to the philosophy of Parmenides (510–450BC), for it was he who argued for an eternal metaphysical Being that contrasted sharply with the transient nature of human beings (Bury and Meiggs 1975; Russell 1996).

When Heidegger spoke of Being, he was referring to no-thing, but to the Parmenidean metaphysical Being, and his choice of *sein*, prefixed by *da* for there, means literally, 'there being'. Heidegger ([1927] 1966) capitalised the word *Dasein*, which is pronounced daa-sine, to distinguish it from the eighteenth-century term *dasein*, pronounced dass-ine, that refers to the actuality of the actual, or 'that one'.

Heidegger developed the concept of Being, as the Being of human beings in the world, but in so doing was careful to avoid the metaphors of science or religion saying:

> The reference to being-in-the-world ... does not imply earthly as opposed to heavenly being, nor the worldly as opposed to the spiritual. For us world does not at all signify beings or any realm of beings but the openness of Being.
>
> (Heidegger [1927] 1996: 252)

Palmer (1969) explained that the term 'world' as in 'Being-in-the-world', meant the world in which humankind is immersed and which is so encompassing that people barely recognise it as they go about their daily business, only becoming aware of it when change occurs. This unconcealing is exemplified by Heidegger ([1927] 1996) when he describes a person using a hammer who uses it quite unconsciously until it breaks, at which time the characteristics, such as the weight of the head, become known to the user. Turning to the role of language in unconcealing, Heidegger is absolutely clear about its role, saying:

> Language is the house of Being. In its home man dwells. Those who think and those who create words are the guardians of this home. Their guardianship accomplishes the manifestation of Being insofar as they bring the manifestation to language and maintain it in language through their speech. ... In its essence, language is not the utterance of the organism ... [but] the clearing-concealing advent of Being itself.
>
> (Heidegger [1927] 1996: 217)

Hans-Georg Gadamer

Hans-Georg Gadamer was born in Marburg in 1900. He entered the university to study philosophy then moved to the University of Freiburg to do a doctorate on Plato. He then worked as assistant to the newly appointed Heidegger and by 1928 completed a second doctorate on Plato under Heidegger's supervision. In 1939 he moved to the University of Leipzig, staying there latterly as rector, until 1947 when he moved to the University of Frankfurt. He accepted a chair at the University of Heidelberg in 1949, retired in 1965, then become emeritus professor, spending the first 20 years of his retirement as visiting professor at many north American universities. He died in Heidelberg on 13 March 2002.

The development of philosophical hermeneutics

Reader (1988) is right to suggest that Gadamer was less radical than Heidegger in his approach to hermeneutics, preferring to pose more humble questions about its scope. One of the reasons for this may be that Gadamer was first and foremost a teacher of philosophy. Reflecting on his philosophical journey, Gadamer said:

> In fact, the rise of my 'hermeneutic philosophy' must be traced back to nothing more pretentious than my effort to be theoretically accountable for the style of my studies and my teaching. Practice came first. For as long ago as I can remember, I have been concerned not to say too much and not to lose myself in theoretical constructions which were not fully made good by experience.
>
> (Gadamer 1997: 16)

But this modest account belies the fact that the Gadamerian corpus numbers over 2,500 items, with much of the work produced just before or after his retirement from the University of Heidelberg in 1965 (Gadamer 1997). To make sense of his contribution, this section will first make the connections between Gadamer, his predecessors and contemporaries, before considering the major strands of his work, which are language, play, prejudice, hermeneutic horizons and the hermeneutic circle (Wolff 1975; Walsh 1996).

Language at the centre of Being

Like Heidegger, Gadamer rejected the view developed by Enlightenment thinkers that, on the one hand, humankind can be studied through empirical observation like the subjects of study in the natural sciences and, on the other, that humankind or their works can be understood by a process of getting inside the author's mind. The reason for this rejection is that, as a Plato scholar, Gadamer located understanding in language, which is maintained through speech:

> Plato was right when he asserted that whoever regards things in the mirror of speech becomes aware of their full and undiminished truth. And he was profoundly correct when he taught that all cognition is only what it is as re-cognition, for 'first cognition' is as little possible as a first word.
>
> (Gadamer [1972] 1976: 25)

Two points emerge from the above. First, in arguing that all cognition is re-cognition, Gadamer dispensed with the Husserlian argument of unsullied data reached through phenomenological reduction. What Gadamer said was that all data have unavoidable linguistic history. Second, if language unconceals Being, then those disciplines where language provides a founda-tion for understanding *must* be epistemologically prior to those that do not. Hekman (1984) noted that in putting language at the centre of Being, Gadamer effectively turned the tables on those from the natural sciences who argued that they had a monopoly on the truth through their 'scientific' methods.

However, another side of removing the inferiority complex felt by some of those who work in the hermeneutic tradition was the moral responsibil-ity for them not to do violence to the text by attempting to dominate it, or appropriate it for their own purposes, for to do that was to do violence to humankind's linguistic heritage. Palmer stated that this means:

> that one does not seek to become master of what is in the text but to become the servant of the text; one doesn't try to observe and see what is in the text, as to follow, participate in, and hear what is said by the text. Gadamer plays on the relationship between listening, belonging and hearing which the word belongingness, *Zugehörigkeit* suggests.
>
> (Palmer 1969: 208)

Palmer noted that the word *Zugehörigkeit*, belongingness, is associated with the word *hören*, which means to harken or to hear, and the word *gehören*, which means to belong to. An example of the way in which older people, their relatives and nurses were helped to belong to the study and the steps taken to hear, but not appropriate, their texts can be found in Chadderton (2003).

The aims and ends of play

Turning to the concept of play, when interviewed by Boyne (1988) Gadamer reminded the interviewer that his background was in classical civilisations and it was from his conception of art that he derived his concept of play. For Gadamer (1997: 101), play was not the state of mind through which the artist approaches their work, nor enjoyment of producing a thing made, not even the freedom to work in a creative manner, but rather the mode of being of the work of art itself and a clue to the way in which mankind comes to understanding. He described it thus:

> If we examine how the word play is used and concentrate on its so called metaphorical senses, we find talk of the play of light, the play of waves, the play of gears and parts of machinery, the interplay of limbs,

the play of forces, the play of gnats, even a play on words. In each case what is intended is a to-and-fro movement which is not tied to any goal that would bring it to an end.

(Gadamer 1997: 103)

The to-and-fro movement is central to understanding play, whether in a child playing with a ball, a team playing in a contest, or a nurse researcher playing with the transcript of an interview (Walsh 1996). In each case the player adopts a different comportment towards the play but in each case new understanding occurs. In the case of the child playing with a ball, it may be that the free mobility of the ball surprises them, which may explain why playing with a rugby ball is seen as good practice for surprises in later life. In respect of the team player in a contest, it is possible that the player will learn something about his performance from the result of the game, and in the case of the nurse researcher it is to be anticipated that they will learn something about the conduct of interviews and the lives of the persons interviewed. In terms of the temporality of understanding, what is certain is that whilst the new understanding will serve the player for a period of time, it will ultimately become out of date and the player will have to engage in more play to understand their new situation.

Ingram (1985) developed the concept of play further by suggesting that in dialogical play, each player approaches the other with their conception of the truth; that in the to-and-fro of the exchange, questions occur from which new truths may emerge. Gadamer ([1960] 1996) considered two charges about the outcome of dialogical play. The first charge is that the resultant new truth is no more than a slippery subjectivity in which anything goes. In answering this charge, Gadamer responded by saying that understanding is neither subjective nor objective but comes from the commonality of language found in the linguistic traditions of the persons engaged in the play. In considering a second charge, that understanding is at best only partial, Gadamer said:

It is obviously correct that no understanding of one person by the other can ever achieve complete coverage of the thing being understood. Here hermeneutical analysis must clear away a false model of understanding and of agreement-in-understanding. An agreement in understanding never means that difference is totally overcome by identity. When one says that one has come to an understanding with someone about something, this doesn't mean that one has absolutely the same position. The German phrase meaning 'one comes to an agreement' *man kommt überein* expresses it very well.

(Gadamer [1972] 1976: 50)

The idea of prejudice

Turning to the idea of prejudice, Gadamer ([1960] 1996) returned to the Middle Ages and the rise of science to explain how the modern concept of prejudice had developed. He argued that scientists and Enlightenment scholars, with their faith in observation and the printed word and their belief in a perfect world, sought to discredit a European society that lived in small communities and close to nature. He added that they would accept no authority other than their own and that the prevailing attitude was the ' ... conquest of mythos by *logos*' Gadamer ([1960] 1996: 273). The result was prejudice being used against traditional ways of understanding including oral history, poetry and folk customs, in fact any route except observation and judgement based on counting.

Gadamer ([1972] 1976) also understood that Heidegger had been right to return to unconcealedness for the truth of Being, but he realised as well that when language unconceals, it brings with it a history and prejudices all of its own. In considering these prejudices Gadamer said:

> It is not so much our judgements as it is our prejudices that constitute our being. This is a provocative formulation, for I am using it to restore to its rightful place a positive concept of prejudice that was driven out of our linguistic use by the French and English Enlightenment. It can be shown that the concept of prejudice did not originally have the meaning we have attached to it. Prejudices are not necessarily unjustified and erroneous, so that they inevitably distort the truth. In fact, the historicity of our existence entails that prejudices, in the literal sense of the word, constitute the initial directedness of our whole ability to experience. Prejudices are biases of our openness to the world. They are simply conditions whereby we experience something.
>
> (Gadamer [1972] 1976: 9)

The idea of prejudice appears to resonate with nurse researchers in three ways. The first is the use of techniques of active listening with prompting and probing during research interviews (Annells 1996; Pascoe 1996), though as Paley (1998) speculated, this may be no more than a reflection of North American humanism and not associated with understanding that language has its history. The second sense is the expression of personal prejudices as part of the research design. Allen (1995) illustrated this by outlining his socio-demographic details in a paper advocating a more critical hermeneutic approach to the provision of healthcare in the United States. Walsh (1996) illustrated his prejudices in a similar way with a personal view of his own work in a review of the elements of Gadamerian hermeneutics. Benner, Tanner and Chesla (1996) made the prejudices of their research team explicit in a six-year study of the nature of knowledge in expert nursing practice. In a third sense, Walters (1996) took the concept of prejudice further when he suggested that prejudices help researchers formulate research questions. Kisiel developed this theme when he argued that hermeneutic research is ecumenical, in that the researcher tries to see the participant's point of view:

> It is true that we may begin by posing an 'academic question' with regard to the text, but the true hermeneutic experience does not begin until we are sufficiently open to permit the text to question us, i.e. to unhinge our prejudices and to suggest its own.
>
> (Kisiel 1985: 9)

This idea has relevance to the ways hermeneutic researchers develop research questions during data collection and analysis. Diekelmann, Allen and Tanner (1989) called this process 'listening to the text'.

Hermeneutic horizons

The term 'hermeneutic horizon' refers to the understanding a person holds about any aspect of their world. Dialogical play with hermeneutic horizons means that when a person views their world – and this includes engaging in dialogue, reading a text or considering pictures, sculpture or buildings (Gadamer [1972] 1976) – the process involves playing with competing versions of the truth a reader brings with them in their language, and the resultant new truth is of its time, which will ultimately be replaced by new truths of their time. In this sense, understanding is a temporary fusion of horizons.

The principal objection to the ideas outlined above is that it is not sufficiently critical of the conditions surrounding understanding (Wolff 1975). Perhaps the greatest critics in this respect are the group of philosophers and social scientists at the University of Frankfurt known as the critical social theorists, a group which includes Jürgen Habermas (1930–), one of Gadamer's former students at the University of Heidelberg. Critical social theory shares some common ground with hermeneutics in that both reject Cartesian dualism, but critical social theorists claim that hermeneutics ignores the power relations in understanding, and that certain interest groups including politics, education and the media have created a reality favourable to their own interests (Allen, Benner and Diekelmann 1986). Critical social theorists also express an interest in changing what they see as domination and repression created by the powerful interest groups (Misgeld 1976). The result of this is that critical social theorists claim some aspects of understanding, because they arise from a different reality, are outside the scope of hermeneutics. Gadamer ([1972] 1976: 21) responded to this claim saying he accepted that understanding necessarily included an appreciation of power relations but to say that there is a reality outside the linguistically constructed world was 'absolutely absurd'.

The hermeneutic circle and zum Stehen kommen

The last of the concepts in Gadamerian hermeneutics is the hermeneutic circle, which is a metaphor for bringing together each of the previous concepts. The hermeneutic circle exemplifies the circularity of play, the temporality of truth, the historicity of language in prejudice and the coming together of interpreter and text in the fusion of horizons. But how does a person know when they have come to a point of understanding? Reference has already been made to *man kommt überein* but Gadamer ([1972] 1976) used a second example, with a military metaphor. He asked, when looking at a battle, whether it was possible to know when an army in flight has come under the command of its officers and is ready to stand and fight the enemy again. He asked was it when the first soldier stopped and turned, or when two soldiers had stopped, or when the last soldier had stopped and turned? (For those who dislike military metaphor, a soccer, rugby football or tennis match seem just as appropriate.) The answer, he suggested, could not be predicted by anyone watching, but is known by all when it happens. This phenomenon of literally coming to a stand, Gadamer ([1972] 1976: 14) said, is expressed in the 'beautiful German word' *zum Stehen kommen*, or coming to understand.

Studies using hermeneutics

The aim of the review is to extend the conversations about the use of hermeneutics that highlight the confusion over conceptual matters and lack of clarity in hermeneutical thinking. The sample of 14 studies was selected for presentation in this book to create dialogue about the ways in which the philosophical underpinnings were described and used and the ways in which findings were presented and discussed. The studies were published between 1992 and 2000 in CINAHL indexed journals.

Review of studies

In the first study, Rather (1992) interviewed 15 registered nurses to determine their lived experience of returning to nursing though a baccalaureate programme. Rather stated that she used Heideggerian phenomenology to provide the philosophical background for her study and supported this claim through the use of primary sources. She used an overtly hermeneutic approach to data collection to help the registered nurses talk about teaching and learning, and analysed the data within the research team using the seven-step Diekelmann, Allen and Tanner (1989) approach. The key findings were expressed in the constitutive pattern *nursing as a way of thinking,* which was made up of nine themes including *teachers who care, teacher as learner, going deeper, gleaning what you can use* and *seeing the big picture.* The findings were presented and discussed within the context of the philosophical underpinnings and the relevant education and role literature.

In her study, Wray (1995) interviewed 10 adults who had suffered family breakdown as a child. Wray stated she used Heideggerian phenomenological hermeneutics to underpin her study and supported this claim through the use of primary sources: she also discussed the differences between Heideggerian and Husserlian phenomenology. Wray analysed her data within a research team using the Diekelmann, Allen and Tanner (1989) approach. She expressed the key findings in the patterns *remembering breakdown, comporting towards breakdown* and *living in thrownness* and explained the meaning of the term 'pattern'. The findings were presented and discussed within the context of Heideggerian hermeneutics and the relevant family breakdown literature.

In their study, Diekelmann and Ironside (1998) used extended interviews with 15 doctoral students to give meaning to the idea of scholarship in doctoral education. The researchers stated that they used Heideggerian phenomenology and Gadamerian hermeneutics as the philosophical foundations of the study and supported their claim through the use of primary sources. Data were analysed within the context of a research team, with the principal findings expressed in the pattern *preserving reading, writing, thinking and dialogue,* which was made up of the themes *writing as technical expertise, writing as thinking, thinking as writing* and *writing as community reflexive scholarship: reawakening dialogue.* The findings were presented with extended exemplars. The doctoral students' experiences were explicated within Gadamerian hermeneutics (Gadamer [1960] 1996). The pattern and themes connected strongly with Heidegger's post-war essays on the nature of thinking (Heidegger [1964] 1996).

In her study, Heliker (1997) stated that she used Heideggerian phenomenology as an approach to help her better understand the quality of care provided for older people in nursing homes. The term 'approach' should not however be taken to mean that Heideggerian phenomenology was just a mere garnish for the work, for having outlined the central ideas of the philosophical underpinnings, Heliker gave a detailed exposition of how Heideggerian phenomenology informed her data collection and analysis. The findings, expressed in the themes *dwelling as remembering, living relatedly* and *Being after loss,* were presented and discussed within the context of the philosophical underpinnings and the relevant nursing homes and gerontology literature. Heidegger's essay on dwelling (Heidegger [1964] 1996) was clearly evident in the themes.

In their study, von Post and Eriksson (1999) used an unusual design to better understand anaesthetic room death and to 'give voice' to suffering and caring in a peri-operative context. The researchers stated that they used

Gadamerian hermeneutics as their philosophical underpinnings and sub-stantiated this claim through the detailed use of primary sources. Of particular note was their discussion of Gadamer's rejection of psychologism and his views on prejudice. The study design was as follows. The first step was to take an essay written by a nurse anaesthetist about the phenomenon of interest. The second step was to interpret the essay in the context of the philosophical underpinnings and express the finding as a complex of prob-lems that included *the patient suffers when the body has let her down* and *the patient suffers when she has been abandoned by the world around her*. The third step was to use the problems to formulate new questions. The fourth step was to use the new questions to further examine the essay. The fifth step was to feed back the interpretations, questions and further inter-pretations to the nurse anaesthetist, who endorsed them. The study design exemplifies the use of dialogical play (Gadamer ([1960] 1996).

The study by Nelms (1996) also used narratives as the data source. In this study, the researcher used stories told by five experienced registered nurses to give meaning to the idea of 'caring presence' in nursing. Nelms did not, however, give a detailed account of her chosen approach of Heideggerian hermeneutics in the methods section of the paper, though she interpreted the registered nurses' stories within the context of seven Heideggerian essays and the relevant caring literature. The findings were expressed in the pattern *care as the presencing of Being*, which was made up of the themes *the timelessness and spacelessness of caring, creating home* and *the call to care as the call of conscience*. The interpretations were then considered by the study participants and endorsed. The pattern and its implications for nursing were discussed within the context of the philo-sophical underpinnings.

In her study, Moloney (1995) stated that she used Heideggerian phenom-enology to elicit 12 older women's experiences of 'being strong', though this was only substantiated by a single reference from a primary source in the methods section of the paper. The findings were expressed in the patterns *surviving, finding strength* and *gathering the memories*. The patterns were made up of nine themes including *living through hard times, putting it behind you, drawing strength from others, being at home* and *looking back over*. However, though the researcher used hermeneutics to guide her data collection and analysis, she did not make reference to them in the discussion of the findings, though she did refer to the relevant gerontology literature.

In her study, Orne (1995), stated that she used Gadamerian hermeneutics to 'inform and guide' her study of the near-death experiences of nine people who had survived cardiac arrest. She substantiated her claim through the use of primary sources. The findings were expressed in the themes *survival: a lived affirmation, survival: an apprehensive plight* and *dying is easy, sur-viving is hard*. However, whilst the researcher used hermeneutics to inform and guide her data collection and analysis, she made only limited use of them in the discussion. What was missing in the paper is the close-coupling of the findings to the philosophical underpinnings.

In his study, Larkin (1998) stated that he used Gadamerian hermeneutics to study the lived experiences of 16 Irish (Gaelic-speaking) palliative care nurses. The researcher substantiated his claim through the use of primary sources. The findings were expressed in the themes *dluchaidreamh* (closeness), *anam chara* (soul-friend), *gramhar* (loving), *aire* (caring) and *sporiad* (spirit). However, whilst the researcher underpinned the study with Gadamerian hermeneutics and used them in the data collection and analysis, he made little reference to them in the presentation and discussion of findings. Where the researcher did use hermeneutics to good effect, however, was in the generation of culturally relevant research questions and the examination of parallel passages from the Celtic literature on death and dying.

In their study, Kerr and McIntosh (1998) stated that they used Heideggerian phenomenology and Gadamerian hermeneutics to underpin their study of the disclosure of infant limb defects to newly delivered mothers. The claim was substantiated through the limited use of primary sources. The researchers interviewed the parents of 29 children born with congenital limb deficiency and expressed the findings in terms of the *parents' feelings and reactions* and *midwives' and doctors' actions* at the point of disclosure and later during the mother's stay in hospital. The researchers stated that the data analysis was guided by Heideggerian and Gadamerian 'principles' but made no reference to the underpinnings in the presentation and discussion of findings.

In her study, Ferguson (1996) stated that she used Gadamerian hermeneutics to 'discover and illuminate' the lived experiences of an unstated number of clinical educators working on a bachelor of nursing programme. The researcher expressed the findings in the themes *developing own teaching style*, *not belonging*, *learn as you go*, *having standards* and *being human*. The researcher supported her claim to have used Gadamerian hermeneutics in an account of the central ideas, but then failed to describe how these had influenced her data collection and analysis. She also failed to make any reference to the philosophical underpinnings, or the education literature, in the presentation and discussion of her findings.

In his study, Walsh (1999) stated that he used Heideggerian phenomenology and Gadamerian hermeneutics to study nurse–patient encounters in psychiatric nursing. The researcher expressed the findings in the themes *Being-with as understanding*, *Being-with as possibility*, *Being-with as careful concern* and *Being-with as listening*. However, whilst Walsh substantiated his use of the philosophical underpinnings through the limited use of primary sources, he did not account for his methodology, preferring instead to refer readers to another of his papers. He then went on to make no further reference to either philosopher in the presentation of his findings and only one unsupported reference to Heidegger in the discussion.

In his study, Smith (1998) stated that he used Gadamerian hermeneutics to study the lives of six problem drinkers. He substantiated his claim through the limited use of primary sources. The findings were expressed in the themes *suffering related to corporeality, suffering in the relational life-world* and *suffering related to time and space*. Smith modified the Diekelmann, Allen and Tanner (1989) approach to data analysis and substantiated these changes in his section on rigour. He then made no further reference to the philosophical underpinnings in the presentation and discussion of findings or in the final section of the paper, where he discussed the implications of his work for research and practice.

Lastly, Vydelingum (2000) stated that he used Heideggerian phenomenology to 'unveil' the experiences of 10 south Asian patients during periods of hospitalisation. The study findings were expressed in the themes *satisfaction, not happy about service, passing through, alone in a crowd* and *we manage somehow*. Vydelingum began by describing the central ideas of Heideggerian phenomenology, largely through secondary sources and with the suggestion that phenomenology provided a method for determining 'concrete' details and 'subjective' experiences. He then failed to make any further reference to the philosophical underpinnings in the presentation and discussion of findings, in the discussion of the methodological issues arising from the study or in his discussion of the implications of the study for nursing practice.

Discussion of the review

In respect of the ways in which the philosophical underpinnings were described and used at key points in the studies above, this connects with two conversations that have relevance within this hermeneutic framework. The first is the argument by Drauker (1999) that whilst it may not be necessary for the researcher to refer to the basic tenets of hermeneutics to remain true to them, there needs to be sufficient detail for readers to understand the contribution that hermeneutics made to the study. The second is the argument by Koch (1994) that rigorous hermeneutical studies state the ontology before following through the epistemology, methodology and method arguments, thus forming a 'decision trail' showing where the study holds its foundations and how those foundations underpin the empirics. In light of this, these studies could be described as follows. Five of the fourteen, Rather (1992), Wray (1995), Heliker (1997), Diekelmann and Ironside (1998) and von Post and Eriksson (1999), adequately described the philosophical foundations at the outset, explicating them at key points. Five others – Nelms (1996), Moloney (1995), Orne (1995), Larkin (1998) and Kerr and McIntosh (1998) – provided minimal information at the outset and subsequently. Four – Ferguson (1996), Smith (1998), Walsh (1999) and Vydelingum (2000) – whilst providing some detail at the outset, failed to give sufficient detail at key points. This observation of the need and ways to clarify and follow through statements of intent can provide useful insight for those planning doctoral education and reviewing papers for publication.

In respect of the ways in which the findings were presented and discussed, this issue connects with the following conversations. First, all the researchers with the exception of von Post and Eriksson (1999) and Kerr and McIntosh (1998) presented their findings as constitutive patterns and themes: the former presented their findings as problems, the latter chose not to categorise their findings. In this context a theme is a 'unit of analysis ... that captures the essence of experience ... creating a web of significance' (DeSantis and Ugarizza 2000: 360), whilst a constitutive pattern expresses the relationship between a group of themes (Diekelmann 1992). The implications of presenting findings as constitutive patterns and themes is that they should be connected, just like a spider's web is connected, to a number of anchor points. In a nursing hermeneutical study these will be the data, the philosophical underpinnings, other relevant literature, and recommendations for further research or practice. Second, Madison (1988) argued that there are nine criteria by which the adequacy of interpretations can be judged. All are relevant, but three are particularly relevant here. They are coherence, comprehensiveness and contextuality, which argue respectively for judgements to be made about the ways in which the interpretations present a unified picture with the philosophical foundations, the ways in which they connect with texts that have an obvious bearing on them and the ways in which they connect with parallel or less obvious texts. Together, these conversations argue for the creation of a connecting conversations approach (Baker and Diekelmann 1994) to the presentation and discussion of findings. In the light of the above, the studies reviewed as follows. A connecting conversations approach was clearly evident in five of the studies: Rather (1992), Wray (1995), Diekelmann and Ironside (1998), Heliker (1997) and von Post and Eriksson (1999). It was less evident in a further four: Nelms (1996), Moloney (1995), Orne (1995) and Larkin (1998), though this last study made excellent connections with parallel texts. It was barely evident in a further four – Kerr and McIntosh (1998), Ferguson (1996), Walsh (1999) and Smith (1998) – and was absent in Vydelingum (2000). These also seem to be issues worthy of consideration by those involved in doctoral education and for those who review papers for publication.

The issues raised above highlight how rigour can be sought, applied and justified in any number of new qualitative methodologies, including the hermeneutic approach illustrated in this chapter, if the researcher is enabled to be accountable through their understanding of the methodological precepts of the framework followed. To reiterate, the key points for searching out rigour from a literature review of hermeneutic studies might include the following:

- the amount of information needed for the reader to understand the study and to follow it through;
- the clarity of progression in a study from ontology to epistemology, methodology and method;
- the presentation of findings as constitutive patterns and themes to create a web of significance;
- the importance of coherence, comprehensiveness and contextuality indicated within Madison's (1988) criteria for the assessment of the adequacy of interpretations.

These, then, are the new guiding forces for those who assess or undertake hermeneutic studies and the argument holds true for other studies in the area of new qualitative methodology. The rigorous pathway, then, should encourage the researcher to state the foundations, follow these through and create connecting conversations between the study and its influences.

References

Allen, D. G. (1995) 'Hermeneutics: Philosophical traditions and nursing practice research', *Nursing Science Quarterly,* 8, 4: 174–82.

Allen, D. G., Benner, P. and Diekelmann, N. L. (1986) 'Three paradigms for nursing research: Methodological implications', in Chinn, P. L., ed., *Nursing Research Methodology: Issues and Implementation*, Rockville, MD: Aspen Publishers.

Alston, W. P. and Nakhnikian, G. (1964) 'Introduction', in Husserl, E. (trans. W. P. Alston and G. Nakhnikian) *The Idea of Phenomenology*, The Hague: Martinus Nijhoff.

Annells, M. (1996) 'Hermeneutic phenomenology: Philosophical perspectives and current use in nursing research', *Journal of Advanced Nursing,* 23: 705–13.

Baker, C. and Diekelmann, N. L. (1994) 'Connecting conversations of caring: Recalling the narrative to clinical practice', *Nursing Outlook,* 42, 2: 65–70.

Benner, P. (1985) 'Quality of life: A phenomenological perspective on explanation, prediction, and understanding in nursing science', *Advances in Nursing Science,* 8, 1: 1–14.

Benner, P., Tanner, C. A. and Chesla, C. A. (1996) *Expertise in Nursing Practice: Caring, Clinical Judgement and Ethics*, New York: Springer Publishing Company.

Boyne, R. (1988) Interview with Hans-Georg Gadamer, *Theory Culture and Society* 5: 25–34.

Burnard, P. (1991) 'A method of analysis of interview transcripts in qualitative research', *Nurse Education Today,* 11: 461–6.

Bury, J. B. and Meiggs, R. (1975) *A History of Greece*, Basingstoke, Hants.: Macmillan.

Chadderton, H. M. (2003) 'Familiar dwelling, fractured dwelling and new dwelling: A Heideggerian–Gadamerian hermeneutic study of the Being of older people in nursing homes', unpublished PhD thesis, University of Wales College of Medicine, Cardiff.

DeSantis, L. and Ugarizza, D. N. (2000) 'The concept of theme as used in qualitative nursing research', *Western Journal of Nursing Research*, 22, 3: 351–72.

Diamond, T. (1992) *Making Gray Gold. Narratives of Nursing Home Care*, Chicago: University of Chicago Press.

Diekelmann, N. L. (1992) 'Learning-as-testing: A Heideggerian hermeneutical analysis of the lived experiences of students and teachers in nursing', *Advances in Nursing Science*, 14, 3: 72–83.

Diekelmann, N. and Ironside, P. (1998) 'Preserving writing in doctoral education: Exploring the concernful practices of schooling, learning, teaching', *Journal of Advanced Nursing*, 28, 6: 1347–55.

Diekelmann, N. L., Allen, D. and Tanner, C. (1989) *The NLN Criteria for Appraisal of Baccalaureate Programs: A Critical Hermeneutic Analysis*, New York: National League for Nursing.

Drauker, C. B. (1999) 'The critique of Heideggerian hermeneutical research', *Journal of Advanced Nursing*, 30: 360–73.

Ferguson, S. (1996) 'The lived experience of clinical educators', *Journal of Advanced Nursing*, 23: 835–41.

Gadamer, H.-G. ([1960]/1996) (trans. J. Weinsheimer and D. G. Marshall) *Truth and Method*, 2nd edn, New York: Continuum (first published 1960).

Gadamer, H.-G. ([1972]/1976) (trans. and ed. D. E. Linge) *Philosophical Hermeneutics*, Berkeley: University of California Press (first published 1972).

Gadamer, H.-G. ([original in English] 1997) 'Reflections on my philosophical journey', in Hahn, L. E., ed., *The Philosophy of Hans-Georg Gadamer*, Chicago: Open Court Publishing Company.

Grant, M. and Hazel, J. (1994) *Who's Who in Classical Mythology*, London: Routledge.

Grondin, J. (1995) *Sources of Hermeneutics*, New York: State University of New York Press.

Gubrium, J. F. (1997) *Living and Dying at Murray Manor* (expanded 2nd edn), Charlottesville, VA: University Press of Virginia.

Gullickson, C. (1993) 'My death as nearing its future: A Heideggerian hermeneutical analysis of the lived experience of persons with chronic illness', *Journal of Advanced Nursing*, 18: 1386–92.

Heidegger, M. ([1927]/1996) (trans. J. Stambough) *Being and Time*, New York: State University of New York Press (first published 1927).

Heidegger, M. ([1964]/1996) (ed. D.F. Krell) *Basic Writings*, London: Routledge (first published 1964).

Hekman, S. (1984) 'Action as text: Gadamer's hermeneutics and the social scientific analysis of action', *Journal for the Theory of Social Behaviour*, 14, 3: 333–53.

Heliker, D. (1997) 'A narrative approach to quality care in long-term care facilities', *Journal of Holistic Nursing* 15, 1: 68–81 (first published 1964).

Highley, B. and Ferentz, T. (1988) 'Esthetic inquiry', in Sarter, B., ed., *Paths to Knowledge: Innovative Research Methods for Nursing*, New York: National League for Nursing.

Husserl, E. ([1907]/1964) (trans. W. P. Alston and G. Nakhnikian) *The Idea of Phenomenology*, The Hague: Martinus Nijhoff.

Ingram, D. (1985) 'Hermeneutics and truth', in Hollinger, R., ed., *Hermeneutics and Praxis*, Indiana: University of Notre Dame Press.

Kerr, S. M. and McIntosh, J. B. (1998) 'Disclosure of disability: Exploring the perspective of parents', *Midwifery,* 14: 225–32.

Kimmerle, H. (1977) Foreword to the German edition, in Schleiermachen, F. D. E. ([1833]/1977) ed. Kimmerle, H. (trans. Duke, J. and Forstman, J.) *Hermeneutics: The Hand-written Manuscripts,* Atlanta, Georgia: Scholars Press.

Kisiel, T. (1985) 'The happening of tradition', in Hollinger, R., ed. *Hermeneutics and Praxis,* Indiana: University of Notre Dame Press.

Koch, T. (1994) 'Establishing rigour in qualitative research: The decision trail', *Journal of Advanced Nursing,* 19: 976–86.

Koch, T. (1995) 'Interpretive approaches in nursing research: The influences of Husserl and Heidegger', *Journal of Advanced Nursing,* 21: 827–36

Krell, D. F. (1996) 'General introduction: The question of being' in Krell, D. F., ed., *M. Heidegger: Basic Writings,* London: Routledge.

Larkin, P. J. (1998) 'The lived experience of Irish palliative care nurses', *International Journal of Palliative Nursing,* 4, 3: 120–6.

Madison, G. B. (1988) *The Hermeneutics of Postmodernity,* Bloomington, IN: Indiana University Press.

McCormick, P. and Elliston, F. A. (1981) *Husserl: Shorter Works* (trans. Jordan, R. W.), Notre Dame, IN: University of Notre Dame Press.

McGrath, A. (1997) *An Introduction to Christianity,* Oxford: Blackwell

Misgeld, D. (1976) 'Critical theory and hermeneutics. The debate between Habermas and Gadamer', in O'Neill, J., ed., *On Critical Theory,* London: Heinemann.

Moloney, M. F. (1995) 'A Heideggerian hermeneutical analysis of older women's stories of being strong', *Image: Journal of Nursing Scholarship,* 27, 2: 104–9.

Morse, J. M., Borttoff, J. L. and Hutchinson S. (1994) 'The phenomenology of comfort', *Journal of Advanced Nursing,* 20, 1: 189–95.

Nelms, T. (1996) 'Living a caring presence in nursing: A Heideggerian hermeneutical analysis', *Journal of Advanced Nursing,* 24: 368–74.

Nelson, J. P. (1996) 'Struggling to gain meaning: Living with the uncertainty of breast cancer', *Advances in Nursing Science,* 18, 3: 59–76.

Omery, A. (1983) 'Phenomenology: A method for nursing research', *Advances in Nursing Science,* 5, 2: 49–63.

Orne, R. (1995) 'The meaning of survival: The early aftermath of near-death experience', *Research in Nursing and Health,* 18: 239–47.

Paley, J. (1997) 'Husserl, phenomenology and nursing', *Journal of Advanced Nursing,* 26: 187–93.

Paley, J. (1998) 'Misinterpretive phenomenology: Heidegger, ontology and nursing research', *Journal of Advanced Nursing,* 27: 817–24.

Palmer, R. E. (1969) *Hermeneutics. Interpretation Theory in Schleiermacher, Dilthey, Heidegger and Gadamer,* Evanston, IL: Northwestern University Press.

Palmer, R. E. (2002) *The Liminality of Hermes and the Meaning of Hermeneutics,* MacMurray College. Accessible at: http://www.mac.edu/~rpalmer.

Pascoe, E. (1996) 'The value to nursing research of Gadamer's hermeneutic philosophy', *Journal of Advanced Nursing,* 24: 1309–14.

Rather, M. L. (1992) 'Nursing as a way of thinking. Heideggerian hermeneutical analysis of the lived experience of the returning RN', *Research in Nursing and Health,* 15: 47–55.

Reader, F. (1988) 'Hermeneutics', in Sarter, B., ed., *Paths to Knowledge: Innovative Research Methods for Nursing*, New York: National League for Nursing.

Rose, P., Beeby, J. and Parker, D. (1995) 'Academic rigour in the lived experience of researchers using phenomenological methods in nursing', *Journal of Advanced Nursing* 21: 1123–9.

Russell, B. (1996) *History of Western Philosophy*, 2nd edn, London: Routledge.

Sandmyer, B. (1988) *Husserl, Edmund 1859–1938. A Schematic Biography*. Accessible at: http://sac.uky.edu%7Ersand1/hus_bio.html (Accessed 22 August 1998).

Santopino, M. (1988) 'The relentless drive to be ever thinner: A study using the phenomenological method', *Nursing Science Quarterly*, 2: 29–36.

Schleiermacher, F. D. E. (1977) (ed. H. Kimmerle) (trans. J. Duke and J. Forstman) *Hermeneutics: The Hand-written Manuscripts* (first published 1833), Atlanta, Georgia: Scholars Press.

Sheehan, T. (1988) 'Heidegger and the Nazis', *The New York Review*, 35, 10: 38–47.

Smith, B. A. (1998) 'The problem drinker's lived experience of suffering: An exploration using hermeneutic phenomenology', *Journal of Advanced Nursing*, 27: 213–22.

Streubert, H. J. (1991) 'Phenomenological research as a theoretical initiative in community health nursing', *Public Health Nursing*, 8, 2: 119–23.

Streubert, H. J. and Carpenter, D. R. (1995) *Qualitative Research in Nursing: Advancing the Humanistic Imperative*, Philadelphia: J.B. Lippincott Company.

Swanson-Kauffman, K. and Schonwald, E. (1988) 'Phenomenology', in Sarter, B., ed., *Paths to Knowledge: Innovative Research Methods for Nursing*, New York: National League for Nursing.

von Post, I. and Eriksson, K. (1999) 'A hermeneutical textual analysis of suffering and caring in the peri-operative context', *Journal of Advanced Nursing*, 30: 983–9.

Vydelingum, V. (2000) 'South Asian patients' lived experience of acute care in an English hospital: A phenomenological study', *Journal of Advanced Nursing*, 32: 100–7.

Walsh, K. (1996) 'Philosophical hermeneutics and the project of Hans-Georg Gadamer: Implications for nursing research', *Nursing Inquiry*, 3: 231–7.

Walsh, K. (1999) 'Shared humanity and the psychiatric nurse-patient encounter', *Australian and New Zealand Journal of Mental Health Nursing*, 8: 2–8.

Walters, A. J. (1996) 'Being a clinical nurse consultant: A hermeneutic phenomenological reflection', *International Journal of Nursing Practice*, 2: 2–10.

Wolff, J. (1975) 'Hermeneutics and the critique of ideology', *Sociological Review* 23: 811–823.

Wray, J. N. (1995) 'Remembering family breakdown: A Heideggerian hermeneutic analysis', *Addictions Nursing*, 7, 2: 54–61.

Chapter 4

Descriptive phenomenology
Life-world as evidence

Les Todres and Immy Holloway

Although phenomenology has a long philosophical heritage, and although its implications for the human sciences have been developing over the course of the past century, the applications of this tradition to research methodology continue to evolve in innovative ways. This chapter will offer something old and something new. It will acknowledge the historical and philosophical foundations of phenomenology, outline some conceptual distinctions that define a phenomenological approach, and finally, illustrate one particular approach to translating these ideas into methodological practice.

The two specific primary concerns of this chapter are to:

- demonstrate the relevance of descriptive phenomenology for health and social care research;
- provide an indication of how this approach continues to evolve.

Towards a focus: philosophical and historical considerations

Two philosophers are central in the development of this approach: Wilhelm Dilthey and Edmund Husserl.

Dilthey considered some of the unique challenges that an acknowledgement of our human participation brings to the subject of psychology and the scientific study of ourselves. He was acutely attuned to how we are embedded in and are part of the psychological life that we are trying to understand, with the result that we cannot say that we are 'objective' as human scientists. Within this perspective, our human interests are always grounded in, and emerging from, a pre-existing involvement in experiential life. It can only be in this sense that our questions are experienced and evaluated as relevant. In our humanness, we are able to evaluate things because we have feelings and purposes; we are able to understand history in a meaningful way because we are historical beings. Dilthey thus called for a *Geisteswissenschaft*, an 'understanding science' that attempts to comprehend the nature of mental life from 'within', rather than from the perspective of an 'outsider', as if we were foreign to ourselves as experiencing beings. Methodologically, Dilthey wishes to begin from a holistic perspective in which human functioning retains its essential characteristic of experiential intelligibility. In this view, a psychology that cannot find a language that discovers the 'I in the thou' (Dilthey in Rickman 1976: 15) has alienated itself from its subject matter.

In emphasising the centrality of human context in understanding psychological life, Dilthey signifies the crucial 'starting point' for an 'understanding science': it begins from what we *already understand* as participants in the human condition:

> If I had no emotions, I could not even begin to understand the love poetry of the Elizabethans, but I can only understand it properly by reading about that period. Once I understand the poems I can gain insight into the thoughts and emotions of people very different from me and this extension of my imaginative insight into human nature will, in turn, help me to understand my own muddled feelings better.
>
> (Dilthey in Rickman 1976: 20)

The process of groping towards a fuller understanding from a less complete understanding is a description of the 'shuttle-cock' movement of what has been called the 'hermeneutic circle'. Such a notion clarifies how understanding proceeds by telling us more about what we already understand, experience and live. In this way, the task of qualitative understanding is to retain continuity with what is already experientially evident and familiar to us as 'commoners'. In considering the participative nature of understanding, Dilthey provides three important ideas, which have become central to the development of phenomenologically oriented research:

- The quest to understand 'more' and 'better' is essentially a qualitative pursuit that requires an 'experience-near' language. It starts with experiences we already understand and expands and deepens these understandings into broader and different contexts through the dialogue with 'otherness'.
- Such understanding proceeds by a mode of analysis in which meaning arises out of relating parts to wholes. That is, we consider how the details and 'evidences' of events contribute to the way in which they fit together with other details and evidences in relation to a larger whole or meaning; correspondingly, the larger whole helps us to see the significance of the details or evidences. This back and forth movement between parts and wholes defines the nature of qualitative understanding. The process of such understanding involves a reflective thematising of the world of meanings that are present in our human engagements and relationships.
- Such a requirement for 'experience-near' evidence and language establishes the need for concrete descriptions of human functioning, and

seeks a disciplined method by which we avoid becoming prematurely abstract in our theorising. Good descriptions of happenings would form the basis from which reflective understandings could proceed.

Edmund Husserl meditated further on the nature of our intimate engagement in experiential life and, out of this, he rigorously developed the subject matter of phenomenological inquiry: the life-world (*Lebenswelt*). Husserl took some guidance from Dilthey's notion of how description is a better starting point than explanation. For Husserl, the concrete affairs (*Sachen*) of everyday life should provide the basis for philosophical reflection.

Although Husserl acknowledged that we always approach situations with our existing understandings, he felt that it is possible for these understandings to become more disciplined and faithful to experiences as they show themselves to us:

> We have to return to the world as it manifests in primordial experience, we must endeavour to find a 'natural' world, the world of immediate experience.
>
> (Kockelmans 1967: 34)

The life-world refers to experiential happenings or occurrences that we live before we know. It is to this 'seamless' stream of living and engagement that we always return as a reference for any qualitative distinctions we make. Distinctions such as 'angry', 'hot' and 'change' only have meaning with reference to the authenticating power of the life-world. This means that such experiential distinctions named as 'hot' and 'angry' are lifted out of a stream of everyday experience – there is essentially no isolated experiential distinction, only what occurs in context, situated in the life-world. This means that if we are to be faithful to the life-world, we describe many things occurring together: where it was, when it was, its 'before' and 'after', how a situation is 'peopled', the meaningful actions, circumstances and sequences. Husserl felt that this was a real starting point for enquiry – that this is how things first come to us, and that later philosophical conclusions and theories can become too abstract if they do not throw light on these beginnings. The group of people that implicitly understand the life-world best are storytellers, who do not separate categories such as mind and body, inner and outer. In order to describe such a richness of happenings in the way things appear together, Husserl asserted that we have to become more naïve in the way we describe the life-world – otherwise we would just assert what we already understood. He held out the possibility that the 'life-world' was a source of evidence beyond our existing understandings and that, if attended to more faithfully, could provide new productive insights.

As questioning beings, to us the life-world often appears to become puzzling in some way. This is what a phenomenon is, something that stands out from the life-world and appears ('asks for attention'). There is a question about its *whatness* – what is it and what makes it what it is? Husserl took this concern with *whatness* from the early Greek philosophers and also wished to take further their deliberations on the quest to articulate 'essences' – the question of something's essential qualities. However, his difference from Plato on this matter was that he did not grant any ultimate objective reality behind the appearances of phenomena. The essences of things do not exist in some ideal mathematical world of which this world is an imperfect modification. Rather the essence of a phenomenon (of what appears), such as sadness, is its distinctive qualities. Husserl was interested in the most valid ways of articulating the essential qualities of phenomena in the way that they appear in relation to their context and how they stand out. This is a meditation on sameness and difference, and on 'good ways' to say this 'sameness' and 'difference'.

There are many controversies that continue to this day about different kinds and levels of Husserl's philosophical quest. However, his lasting contribution to a phenomenologically oriented approach to qualitative research lies in the following two goals:

- to use the 'life-world' as a source of evidence for our enquiries;
- to articulate, not a theory, but good ways of describing the 'whatness' of a phenomenon as it appears, so that we may better understand its nature.

There are many other philosophical distinctions that Husserl and other phenomenological philosophers have made, such as the 'intentionality' of consciousness, the phenomenological reduction, and imaginative variation, all of which have been used when translating this approach into an empirical research methodology. But the above two goals concerning 'life-world' and 'whatness' provide an adequate direction for a distinctive application to phenomenologically oriented empirical research.

One approach to how this philosophy has informed research practice

There have been a number of ways in which phenomenological philosophy has influenced the development of empirical research (Polkinghorne 1989; Moustakas 1994; Von Eckartsberg 1998, Van Kaam, 1959). The approach that we wish to illustrate in this chapter, that of descriptive phenomenology, is one that has arisen out of psychology and that has stayed fairly close to Husserl's emphasis on the 'life-world' and the task to describe and articulate the 'whatness' of a phenomenon as it 'comes to appear' in experienced happenings.

A psychologist who has been pivotal in translating philosophical phenomenology into an empirical–phenomenological method that is descriptive in emphasis is Amedeo Giorgi, who developed his approach at Duquesne University in Pittsburgh, USA. He had steeped himself in the writings of Husserl and Merleau-Ponty and was particularly struck by their criticisms of psychology achieving scientific status by imitating the physical sciences. Giorgi developed this theme by writing a ground-breaking book, *Psychology as a Human Science,* in which he offered alternative criteria for human science research that could honour the study of human experience in terms more consistent with its subject matter (Giorgi 1970). These alternative criteria focused on the concern to articulate the qualitative meaning of experiential phenomena rather than their measurement. Giorgi, and colleagues and students at Duquesne University, developed this approach in applied contexts and illustrated it in relation to a number of empirical studies on experiential phenomena, such as the nature of learning something new (Giorgi 1975), the experience of being criminally victimised (Fischer and Wertz 1979), and the phenomenon of self-deception (Fischer 1985).

In developing descriptive phenomenology as an empirical research approach, Giorgi distinguished between Husserl's philosophical phenomenology and the possibility of scientific phenomenology as it may be applied to research practice in the human sciences (Giorgi 2000). The relationship between the philosophy and the scientific practice was articulated as follows:

> Phenomenological philosophy is a foundation for scientific work; it is not the model for scientific practice. The insights of the philosophy have to be mediated so that scientific practices can be performed.
>
> (Giorgi 2000: 4)

Based on modifications of the contributions of Giorgi (1997) and Churchill and Wertz (2001), we would like to offer here four stages of empirical–phenomenological research as a scientific practice that is informed by phenomenological philosophy:

1   Articulating an experiential phenomenon of interest for study.
2   Gathering descriptions of others' experiences that are concrete occasions of this phenomenon.
3   Intuiting and 'testing' the meanings of the experiences.
4   Writing a 'digested' understanding that cares for different readers and purposes.

We will present each of these stages in some detail, paying attention to some of the practical considerations involved, and illustrating where appropriate with examples from practice.

Articulating an experiential phenomenon of interest for study

At this stage, researchers acknowledge and make explicit their initial interest and agenda. As researchers within an 'understanding science' approach, we acknowledge our human embeddedness and participation in experiential life. This includes a sensitivity to our own historical, professional and community contexts. Our beginning understandings about an area of interest are intimately informed by significances of which we are part: perhaps a community of scholars focused on developing a topical area through writing and research, perhaps some gaps and unanswered questions that stand out in relation to the literature, perhaps a burning personal question grounded in personal and social history, perhaps something significant about what is happening at this moment in time. What initially motivates our enquiries is thus part of this natural world of everyday engagements and contexts in which we participate.

The phenomenologically informed researcher acknowledges this but needs to do some more disciplined work on the formulation of the research question before the research can proceed. The value of acknowledging existing engagements and interests is that it locates the topic and subject manner in a general way that can connect to everyday human concerns and directions. So, for example, one of the authors was interested in a long historical debate in the literature about the nature of self-insight in psychotherapy. However, he took direction for his study not only from his concern to 'speak to' this debate, but also from a concern to help his students practise psychotherapy in a more thoughtful way. So, his interest was not just academic, but also practical. He found it useful, as a starting point for articulating the research question, to make his interests and engagements with the topic more explicit, as follows:

> For a long time I have been fascinated by how understanding oneself more, one's motives, thoughts, feelings, and position can lead to a greater sense of felt freedom. Socrates talked about this, Freud talked about this, and I and friends, family and clients all have had this experience at one time or another: that certain kinds of self-insight appeared to carry a greater sense of freedom. The rationale of a particular cultural practice in the twentieth century, psychotherapy, is based on this possibility: an interpersonal situation which is specifically set up to help people feel freer and act more coherently in their personal lives through self-insight. So as a practising psychotherapist, I was interested in self-insight, felt freedom and the practice of psychotherapy. Although different theories had certain explanations of what self-insight is, very few were able to let go of their particular theoretical framework (e.g. 're-organising psychic energy', or 'cognitive restructuring') and describe what was occurring in a more naïve and context-rich way. Being familiar

with phenomenology and existentialism I was interested in the question: what is the nature of the kind of psychotherapeutic self-insight that leads to a greater sense of freedom? ... My concern in attempting to elucidate these questions is connected to another concern: to help myself and other health practitioners to practise psychotherapy in a more thoughtful and helpful manner so that our clients benefit. I was thus interested in this discovery-oriented research in order to help myself and other practitioners to learn for the sake of acting.

(Todres 2000: 43)

Gathering descriptions of others' experiences that are concrete occasions of this phenomenon

At this stage, researchers discipline their preconceptions in such a way as to formulate an 'experience-near' question that can invite life-world descriptions from others. This move goes back to Husserl's concern that enquiry should be grounded in the life-world. A term like 'self-insight' may be a useful theoretical construct, but what actual experiences does it refer to? Is it the best word for important experiences of this kind or is its meaning excessively contaminated with theory and different schools of thought? There are two problems with just accepting this word without question as a point of departure: it can impose a preconceived theoretical framework on the direction of the researcher's enquiry, and it is a word that is not 'experience-near' enough for research respondents to relate to when identifying a related experience that they have lived through.

Researchers at this phase do what it takes to become as open-minded as possible by disciplining their preconceptions. In spite of the theoretical frameworks that may have been achieved historically, and in spite of their own interests and engagements, the researchers 'stand back' and 'go back to basics' by asking an open-ended phenomenological question in the following form: *What* is the *experience* to which the word or topic ('self-insight') may refer? They do not know in advance whether this experience exists – they will find this out from the evidence of people's descriptions of life-world events. But they need to find an open-ended, 'experience-near' question that invites respondents to speak about a related phenomenon as real to the respondents as an experience that they have personally lived through.

Husserl has provided helpful pointers in formulating such an experience-near question that may invite life-world descriptions, and this centres on his understanding that all experience is situated. The technical term for this is 'intentionality'. It means that consciousness and experience is never just an 'inner' experience but is interactional and refers to relationships in the world. So, if I am asking you to describe a life-world experience, a good way of asking this is to say: 'Can you describe a *situation* in which you ...?'

In this way, the respondent is invited to describe happenings, the story of the phenomenon, where, when, with whom, and then feelings, meanings, and all of the narrative context that is the stream of experiencing from which a phenomenon stands out.

In the case of the study of self-insight in psychotherapy, such a process of 'standing back' and the concern to become more faithful to the characteristics of the 'life-world' resulted in a realisation that the term 'self-insight' could refer to a whole range of actual experiences, including experiences that were both unhelpful and helpful. This resulted in a more refined question about a particular kind of self-insight that could be central to psychotherapy and that could be expressed in experience-near ways. So this author arrived at a surprising but interesting question that had not been dealt with in those terms in the literature. He made the following request of relevant respondents: 'Describe a situation in psychotherapy in which you saw something or understood something which carried with it a greater sense of freedom.'

When, in a pilot study, the author asked respondents a question about 'self-insight', a number did not know what he was talking about. When he later asked the same respondents the above question, most were able to identify a relevant experience of this kind, which they had lived through. The rest were able to say something like: 'I understand what you are asking for, but I do not have an experience of this kind.'

There are different ways that a researcher can gather experience-near, life-world descriptions by others, such as interviews, verbal testimony, written protocols, media representations and even artworks. The central spirit of these first two stages, however, is to find a way of naming the experiential phenomenon of interest in such a manner that can be asked in an open-minded way: *What* is it and *how* does it *live* in life-world experiences? Such a focus results in *descriptions* of experiential happenings that can function as evidence for further understanding and reflection.

Intuiting and 'testing' the meanings of the experiences

Husserl and descriptive phenomenology would say that the possible depth and meaning of a descriptive account of an experience can go beyond the conclusions and interpretations of the one having the experience. The phenomena that people live have some generalisable properties: there is something about 'anger' that we can recognise in Joe, Sally and also Peter – there is something about the properties that makes us feel there is something distinctive about 'anger'. In this sense, a description of experience is an 'open text' that can lead to insights in more general ways than just this specific occasion. The 'thereness' of the experience can lead to transferable insights about the phenomenon, constituting a thematic pattern amongst a number of experiential examples. As researchers who are human beings, we participate in the life-world (in part/whole engagements) and as such, can understand what something may be like as an experience – we do not just have 'empty words' from others' descriptions, but 'have' how these words refer to a whole experiential world of significances. We can reflect on these significances and check out whether these significances are verified by various details of an experience. This is what makes phenomenological analysis possible and the quest to articulate transferable meanings. So, this stage has as its goal the articulation of transferable meanings that can tell us something 'more' and interesting about the phenomenon. This is not just a presentation in similar or other words of the 'voices' of the research respondents. Rather, the descriptions by the research respondents serve as a 'window' for forms of analysis that, at a certain point, move beyond the expressions of the respondents, in order to elucidate possible meanings in a more general way. The technical details of this goal may practically proceed as follows: A number of descriptions of experience are reflected on to reveal transferable meanings that are relevant to clarifying the phenomenon under study. Giorgi and others have recommended some stages of analysis that assist in intuiting and expressing general meanings in a disciplined way and try to be faithful to the details and 'evidences' of the particular descriptive accounts (Giorgi *et al.* 1975; Giorgi 1985; Wertz 1983; Anstoos 1985; Von Eckartsberg 1998; Fischer 1998).

Although the technical details of these stages can be divided into three or more phases, the procedure essentially aids the task of intuition and reflection by providing different occasions for meanings to cohere through different factual variations. The procedure is designed to ensure that the details of individual experiences intimately contribute to an articulation of a level of generality considered to be relevant. For example, in a study of the experience of the transition to motherhood, Hartley (personal communication) considered a number of examples where 'planning' entered life in a much more insistent way. Here is an example of an actual detail from the description of a respondent:

> Normally if I wanted to go anywhere I'd get up, get dressed and go out whereas now it's get up, get 'A' fed, bathed, get the car-seat out, get his change bag out, check his nappy, then by the time you've done all that you think, I'll just change his nappy one more time before we go out. Then you've got to sort of get him down to the car, it's just a lot of hassle as opposed to literally getting up, getting yourself ready and going out.

There are particular qualities to this experience that can be named in general and were expressed as follows:

> Prior to motherhood, going out was a spontaneous activity involving minimal preparation. However, with a baby to organise, outings have

to be planned in advance and the logistics are time-consuming and complicated.

The intuition of transferable meanings, such as the quality and kind of planning that enters the life of a new mother, occurs through the researcher exposing him/herself to a number of variations of experience. They may not use the word 'planning' but this term may 'come to' the researcher as he/she looks for transferable qualities. This is the back and forth movement between emerging themes and specific details. In this process, he/she may realise that the word 'planning' does not say it well enough. So in the example above, the details such as 'car seat' and 'changing nappy one more time' indicate a kind of anticipatory care to the planning. So, in testing a more distinctive theme of planning with anticipatory care, we need to go to other examples, perhaps from other mothers, to see whether this emerging meaning can be further refined and tested from actual descriptive evidences. Such intuition and articulation of meanings involves a kind of disciplined imagination in which we are open to the meaning coming to us but with the requirement that it is not just a poetic flight, in that it can be justified by the details of the actual descriptions. The validity lies in the judgement by others of whether the researcher puts together the meanings in a good and helpful way, and whether the meanings adequately capture the sense of the details.

Writing a 'digested' understanding that cares for different readers and purposes

This stage involves two concerns: one scientific and one communicative. The scientific concern cares for the phenomenon and the experiences of the research respondents; the communicative concern cares for the readers of the research document and for the purposes to which the research may be put.

The scientific concern

The intuition and articulation of essences is the attempt to move from specific individual experiences to a level of generality that rigorously expresses the phenomenon studied in a coherent way. The aim is to establish what is typical of the phenomenon and to express such typicality in an insightful and integrated manner. Husserl's emphasis on essences required finding meanings that were invariant across the specific situations. We do this all the time although often unconsciously: finding patterns which we then test out to see whether the pattern still holds in other situations. To describe what is essentially typical across cases has also been referred to as the 'general structure' of the phenomenon and has been further defined as follows:

To describe the structure is to describe how the elements of a phenomenon function constitutively, how they interrelate to form the unity of the experience.

(Reed 1987: 102)

Husserl discussed various levels of generality that were possible, for example, trying to find a meaning about a phenomenon that is universally applicable so that the statement is true about all cases. This is perhaps most possible in the physical sciences where 'laws' can be found as invariant across events. However, in the human sciences, where complex human experiences straddle the variations of unique individuals, culture, language and many other contexts, 'essences' are never context-free. The level of generality or invariance in human science is thus not necessarily universally applicable, but applies within similar contexts:

Psychologists are more interested in essences that are context related, or relevant for typical situations or typical personalities and so on, rather than the universal as such.

(Giorgi 1985: 50)

Practically, intuiting and expressing 'invariances' across cases means that one is carefully considering the role and status of the variations within the structure. This involves both intuition and logic (as in other sciences), as one is 'holding' in one's imagination both the 'digested' understanding of the phenomenon as it was revealed by the various descriptions, as well as an openness to have this understanding changed by further details. The writing of the 'general structure' reflects all this and formulates:

an integrative statement that conveys the coherent structure of the psychic life under consideration – its various constituents (e.g. temporal phases) and their relations within the whole.

(Churchill and Wertz 2001: 252)

For example, in a study on the phenomenology of forgiveness and reconciliation, Fow (1996) provided a summarised structure of 'forgiving another', describing important essential features that make sense of the cases he studied. One essential feature concerned how an individual achieved a change of perspective about a perception of being personally violated. So, one of the 'invariant essences' of this experience was that a change in perspective was achieved. However, this change of perspective was achieved in a number of different ways and Fow's general structure articulated these variations as a means of clarifying what was invariant as well as what was variant. He highlighted at least three ways in which the essential feature could occur: by identifying with the other, by understanding something more about the circumstances of the other, and by taking the action less personally within a larger philosophical framework. These three variations may overlap but articulate different nuances of the achievement of a change of perspective. The essential structure of a phenomenon cannot thus be clarified without showing how its invariant themes 'live out' in variant possible ways. The 'scientific concern' of the writing thus enhanced credibility by elaborating on each of the invariant themes and by giving examples of how they took place with reference to the particular experiences of research respondents. In his study on forgiveness and reconciliation, Fow followed his sum- marised structure by elaborating on each of the themes with examples from his respondents. Thus, in a section entitled 'the movement towards forgive- ness', he quoted excerpts from Patti's experience as well as Jane's experience in order to clarify both common themes and their possible variations. Sometimes the variations themselves cluster into three or four kinds of vari- ations; we generalise where it is helpful and the phenomenological researcher needs to make judgements about whether the expression of essences and their variations are coherent and justified from the life-world evidence. Ashworth (2000) referred to this kind of validity as 'descriptive adequacy', by which he meant that the 'description achieved is not merely a consequence of the prejudices that were brought to the research at the start' (2000: 149), but that the description has been intimately informed by the 'evidence' of the 'life-world' happenings. In concrete terms, we may ask whether the researcher has paid enough attention to these 'scientific con- cerns' so that, in writing up his/her 'digested understanding', he/she has given enough examples to enable the reader to see what the researcher saw.

The communicative concern

In considering the readers of the research document and the purposes to which the research may be put, it may often be useful to preface the writing of one's digested understanding by making it explicit whom the writing is intended for, and something about the intended style and level of writing. For example, in the previously cited study on self-insight in psychotherapy, Todres (2000) made explicit the following intentions:

> In writing my description of therapeutic self-insight I was thus pre-
> occupied with this question of 'learning for acting' and its implications
> for how my discoveries would be presented. I was not sure in advance
> what this mode of presentation was, but considered the following ini-
> tial signposts:
> - It will be more than a definition or series of statements about ther-
>   apeutic self-insight.
> - It will tell us something that connects with universal human quali-
>   ties so that the reader can relate personally to the themes.

- It will tell a story which readers can imagine in a personal way.
- It will attempt to contribute to new understanding about therapeutic self-insight.
- It will not attempt to exhaust the topic but will attempt to allow it to be seen more clearly: like shining a light which increases the reader's sense of contact with this phenomenon without fully possessing it.

(Todres 2000: 43)

This is an example of just one possible variation in presenting findings. In this case, Todres supplemented the presentation of the general structure with a more narrative account, which attempted to facilitate empathic understanding in readers. His communicative concern emphasised an aesthetic focus (Todres 1998), which attempted to communicate the 'thickness' or richness of the experience. There is a judgement here as to the kinds and levels of communication that would be helpful for different purposes. Different phenomenological researchers have 'cut the cake' in different ways. For example, Moustakas (1994) addresses a number of different levels of generality in presenting findings and includes examples that differentiate between a number of different technical possibilities: a textural description, a structural description, a composite structural description and a textural–structural synthesis. The danger with too many kinds and levels of presentation is that they can be repetitive and reduce rather than enhance the experience of understanding in readers. An important consideration in this regard is how to retain the richness and texture of individual experiences when formulating a level of description that applies more generally and typically.

With regard to the communicative concern of our writing, the literary traditions are helpful in contributing useful purposes and practices. For example, Booth (1987) in his book *The Rhetoric of Fiction* provides helpful directions for more self-aware forms of writing, which can deepen their aesthetic appeal and engage the 'hearts' of readers in an invitational rather than an authoritarian manner.

In an article entitled 'Making phenomenology accessible to a wider audience', Halling (2002) addresses allied communicative concerns. He considers how phenomenological research could be presented differently in order to accentuate its value to clinicians, policy makers and ordinary people. His recommendations include a consideration of the issues involved in writing at different levels:

Who is the audience for our research reports? Is it fellow phenomenologists, mainstream researchers, a broad range of readers from varied disciplines, practitioners who are working with patients, educated lay persons interested in understanding some aspect of their own lives better, or some combination of the above?

(Halling 2002: 30–1)

In conclusion to this section on writing a digested understanding of the phenomenon studied, we would like to venture that a good general guideline is to consider both the scientific and the communicative concerns in your writing. In this regard, it may be useful to think of the phenomenological researcher as a mediator between the 'voices' and experiences of the research respondents and the broader community of interested people.

The relevance of descriptive phenomenology for health and social care research

There is increasing reference in the health and social care arenas to the importance of understanding users, patients and clients of services (Heyman 1995; Bray *et al.* 2000; Rose 2001). For example, in the United Kingdom, clinical governance policies (Department of Health 1998) emphasise the need for involving patients in feedback and decision making. Patient satisfaction questionnaires, focus groups and patient representation on ethics committees and other relevant decision-making bodies have become the order of the day. At the same time, technological advances have brought the issue of 'quality of life' to the fore as one of the central constituents of health and social well-being. The exhortation for research methodologies in health and social care is to find meaningful and adequate ways to present the experiences of users and highlight the 'quality of life' issues. The great danger here is one of superficiality and of not meaningfully reflecting the experiences of patients and clients 'on the ground'.

It is with regard to these dangers that we would like to consider the difference between research that presents users' *views* and research that is based on descriptions of users' *life-worlds*.

Imagine that we wish to better understand what happens when a patient is given a diagnosis he/she was not expecting. Using a descriptive phenomenological approach that focuses on their life-world, we would ask patients who have had this experience to describe as fully as possible the story of the happening, the events in sequence, their interactions, the 'before' and 'after', their thoughts, feelings and behaviours – all that goes into the meaning of the experience for them. The value of such life-world description is that it provides sources of information that may not have been anticipated by either the respondent or the researcher. It does not depend on the ability of the respondent to come up with already formulated views or articulate generalisations. It provides descriptions of the lived experience on which the views may be based, and as such, provides important references for what the views *mean* in specific terms, and how the experience was lived.

Phenomenological researchers thus often encounter the situation where users' 'views' change and deepen as the respondent describes their experience in greater detail. Respondents then sometimes say that this process helped them feel more 'heard' than if they were required to come up with ready-made answers and conclusions. The concerns that arise are often more nuanced and help to form transferable meanings that are more novel and helpful than the reification of an already formulated opinion. So, for example, one respondent may have expressed the view that the doctor did not tell her the truth. We could imagine this theme becoming a reified category and find a number of cases in which the doctor 'did not tell the truth'. But what is the experience that this view refers to? This is a life-world question. And we may find that when the respondent describes the situation, we begin to understand what 'not telling the truth' means. We may find, for example, that a story emerges of confusions and missed opportunities in very specific places rather than a simple 'not telling the truth'. Such detailed descriptions then have the benefit of informing insightful and nuanced directions such as 'confusion of the patient occurred most when provided with a report of a special investigation which came out as normal'. How to deal with the communication of the complexity of special investigations then becomes a much more 'lively' and informative issue than the earlier reified view.

A strong indication that a life-world methodology is entering mainstream health and social care services is evidenced by the UK's National Health Service modernisation agency, which is adopting a methodology of 'discovery interviews' where detailed guidance is given to health and social care practitioners in how to elicit experiential descriptions from users in order that services may be improved (Wilcock *et al.* 2003).

In highlighting the relevance of descriptive phenomenology for health and social care, we would like to conclude with a remark about 'evidence'. The notion of 'evidence-based practice' has become a topical ideology in current health and social care policies and practice (Dawes *et al.* 1999). The challenge, given our analysis, is to broaden the notion of evidence to encompass the human sciences in which 'qualitative' evidence can become an important reference and methodological goal.

An indication of current innovation in theory and methodology

Phenomenology has coalesced with qualitative research in both generic and specific ways. The term is sometimes used in a generic way to include a wide range of qualitative approaches, suggesting that it refers to any sensibility in research that is respectful of reflecting the complexity of human experience in a qualitative way. On the other hand, Giorgi (1997) is very specific about the boundaries of phenomenological research and presents some criteria of inclusion that are closely informed by Husserl's thoughts. They outline an approach that requires a consideration of 'essences', intentionality, life-world, intuition, phenomenological reduction and imaginative variation. The burgeoning complexity of this field can be understood when one considers how

Husserl's writings were important for a whole generation of philosophers and social theorists after him, from existentialists to hermeneuticists, critical theorists, feminists and postmodern deconstructionists. Phenomenology has influenced the development of ethnomethodology (Turner 1974; Button 1991) narrative research (Josselson and Lieblich 2001) and mindful inquiry (Bentz and Shapiro 1998).

As one indication of current innovation, we would like to highlight a direction taken by one of the authors that attempts an integration (Todres 1999) of descriptive phenomenology with Gendlin's philosophy of the implicit (Gendlin 1991). There are two emphases here, a theoretical one that offers a re-evaluation of the goal of descriptive phenomenology to articulate 'essences', and a practical direction, which considers the value of Gendlin's procedure of 'focusing' for interviewing.

Gendlin has been in dialogue with the phenomenological tradition for many years. As early as 1973 he was concerned that the notion of 'essence' could be applied in such a way that we turn lived experiences that are ongoing and always 'greater' and 'more' than any way we can formulate them into linguistic 'summations' that are too static and abstract (Gendlin 1973). Gendlin was concerned that what is 'most general' about experienced phenomena can never be the final thing said about that phenomenon. Todres (2004) has recently taken up some of these considerations in order to re-evaluate the goal of descriptive phenomenology. He expresses this re-evaluation in the following way:

> There is always a 'more' in living and we cannot say this all at once and finally. The phenomenon 'anger' can be understood in richer ways but each new word or phrase is not an 'essence' but rather a 'gathering'. It is a gathering that is instructional (rather than summative), as if to say: when the 'explosiveness' of anger is named, see how 'anger' in the contexts you are interested in is better understood and leads to even further productive understandings and meaningful connections. The word 'explosiveness' is thus a 'lived platform' and bridge rather than an 'essence'.

> (Todres 2004: 52)

Such an emphasis would reframe the idea of 'essence' to be that of an 'authentic productive linguistic gathering': 'authentic' in that the enquiry is based on life-world descriptions; 'productive' in that the findings are expressed in a way that allows readers themselves to engage in dialogue with the 'aliveness' of the phenomenon that the words point to, and to take the understandings further in multiple ways; 'linguistic' in that the presentation in descriptive phenomenology is in the form of explicit language rather than music or some other presentational art form; 'gathering' in that the expression of findings is not considered absolute nor merely arbitrary. Instead, the findings are relevant and truthful offerings by the phenomenological researcher that carry transferable insights as potential 'platforms' for others.

The practical application that emerges from Gendlin's thoughts addresses the age-old problem of how to elicit a description of experiencing that exceeds our conscious reflections. The phenomenologist Merleau-Ponty (1962) clarified the philosophical framework for this challenge when he wrote that the 'lived is greater than the known'. Good descriptions of human experience often carry what is implicit in the experience, for example, the absence of certain words can say just as much as what is said. But let us take this further. Imagine that we are interviewing Mandy about her experience of homelessness. We can see that at times she struggles to find the right words to convey the complexity of her situation. Her 'felt sense' of her situation is the reference she uses when deciding whether some words 'fit' or not. She knows how to recognise when a certain way of saying something is better than another way of saying it.

This example indicates that, as human beings, we often 'dip' into this more implicit sense of our situation as a whole and try to make some of this explicit in words. In his experiential method of focusing, Gendlin (1996) provides some guidelines relevant to psychotherapy that may also be relevant for qualitative interviewing. The differences between psychotherapeutic interviewing and interviewing for the purpose of qualitative research may be important and Todres is engaged in attempting to apply this approach in practice. The task is to help interviewees honour and 'speak from' the implicit 'felt sense' of their situation so that 'more' of the depth of the experience can be articulated. This is a complex project and the scientific, therapeutic and ethical issues that are involved require careful thought. We hope that we have just indicated enough of these innovations to demonstrate that descriptive phenomenology is still 'young' in both its theory and practice and that exciting challenges remain and call for creative and thoughtful contribution.

Concluding thoughts

This chapter has sought to offer enough of the range and depth of descriptive phenomenology in order that readers may:

- understand the value of exploring the historical and philosophical underpinnings of descriptive phenomenology;
- appreciate its practical potential for application by detailing one way of formulating its methodological aims and stages;
- ponder its potential for possible relevance to health and social care research within their own areas of interest and practice;
- be invited to contribute to ongoing innovations to this living tradition of approach and practice.

Clarifying the life-world is something we have all been engaged in since the time we could speak. Descriptive phenomenology is just a more disciplined and reflective way of doing this.

References

Anstoos, C. M. (1985) 'The structure of thinking in chess', in Giorgi, A., ed., *Phenomenology and Psychological Research*, Pittsburgh, PA: Duquesne University Press.

Ashworth, P. (2000) 'The descriptive adequacy of qualitative findings', *The Humanistic Psychologist*, 28, 1–3: 138–52.

Bentz, V. M. and Shapiro, J. J. (1998) *Mindful Inquiry in Social Research*, London: Sage Publications.

Booth, W. (1987) *The Rhetoric of Fiction*, Harmondsworth, London: Peregrine Books.

Bray, J. N., Lee J., Smith, L. L. and Yorks, L. (2000) *Collaborative Inquiry in Practice: Action, Reflection and Meaning Making*, Thousand Oaks, CA: Sage Publications.

Button, G. (1991) *Ethnomethodology and the Human Sciences*, Cambridge: Cambridge University Press.

Churchill, S. D. and Wertz, F. J. (2001) 'An introduction to phenomenological research in psychology', in Schneider, K. J., Bugental, F. T. and Pierson, J. F., eds, *The Handbook of Humanistic Psychology: Leading Edges in Theory, Research and Practice*, London: Sage Publications.

Department of Health (1998) *A First Class Service: Quality in the New NHS*, London: HMSO.

Dawes, M., Davies, P., Gray, A., Mant, J., Seers, K. and Snowball, R. (1999) *Evidence-based Practice: A Primer for Health Care Professionals*, Edinburgh: Churchill Livingston.

Fischer, C. T. and Wertz, F. J. (1979) 'Empirical phenomenological analysis of being criminally victimized', in Giorgi, A., Smith, D. and Knowles, R., eds, *Duquesne Studies in Phenomenological Psychology*, Pittsburgh, PA: Duquesne University Press.

Fischer, C. T. (1998) 'Being angry revealed as self-deceptive protest: An empirical phenomenological analysis', in Valle, R., ed., *Phenomenological Inquiry in Psychology: Existential and Transpersonal Dimensions*, New York: Plenum Press.

Fischer, W. F. (1985) 'Self-deception: An existential–phenomenological investigation into its essential meanings', in Giorgi, A, ed., *Phenomenology and Psychological Research,* Pittsburgh, PA: Duquesne University Press.

Fow, N. R. (1996) 'The phenomenology of forgiveness and reconciliation', *Journal of Phenomenological Psychology*, 27, 2: 219–33.

Gendlin, E. T. (1973) 'Experiential phenomenology', in Natanson, M., ed., *Phenomenology and the Social Sciences*, Evanston, IL: Northwestern University Press.

Gendlin, E. T. (1991) 'Crossing and dipping: Some terms for approaching the interface between natural understanding and logical formation', in Galbraith, M. and Rappaport, W. J., eds, *Subjectivity and the Debate over Computational Cognitive Science*, Buffalo State University of New York: Center for Cognitive Science.

Gendlin, E. T. (1996) *Focusing Oriented Psychotherapy: A Manual of the Experiential Method*, London: The Guildford Press.

Giorgi, A. (1970) *Psychology as a Human Science: A Phenomenologically Based Approach*, New York: Harper and Row.

Giorgi, A. (1975) 'An application of phenomenological method in psychology', in Giorgi, A., Fischer, C. and Murray, E., eds, *Duquesne Studies in Phenomenological Psychology*, Pittsburgh, PA: Duquesne University Press.

Giorgi, A. (1985) *Phenomenology and Psychological Research*, Pittsburgh, PA: Duquesne University Press.

Giorgi, A. (1997) 'The theory, practice and evaluation of the phenomenological method as a qualitative research procedure', *Journal of Phenomenological Psychology*, 28, 2: 235–60.

Giorgi, A. (2000) 'The status of Husserlian phenomenology in caring research', *Scandinavian Journal of Caring Science*, 14: 3–10.

Giorgi, A., Fischer, C., and Murray, E., eds, (1975) *Duquesne Studies in Phenomenological Psychology*, (Vol. 2). Pittsburgh, PA: Duquesne University Press.

Halling, S. (2002) 'Making phenomenology accessible to a wider audience', *Journal of Phenomenological Psychology*, 33, 1: 19–38.

Heyman, B. (1995) *Researching User Perspectives on Community Health Care*, London: Chapman and Hall.

Josselson, R. and Lieblich, A. (2001) 'Narrative research and humanism', in Schneider, K. J., Bugental, F. T. and Pierson, J. F., eds, *The Handbook of Humanistic Psychology: Leading Edges in Theory, Research and Practice*, London: Sage Publications.

Kockelmans, J. J., ed., (1967) *Phenomenology: The Philosophy of Edmund Husserl and its Interpretation*, New York: Doubleday and Company.

Merleau-Ponty, M. (1962) *The Phenomenology of Perception* (trans. Colin Smith), London: Routledge and Kegan Paul.

Moustakas, C. (1994) *Phenomenological Research Methods*, London: Sage Publications.

Polkinghorne, D. E. (1989) 'Phenomenological research methods', in Valle, R. S. and Halling, S., eds, *Existential Phenomenological Perspectives in Psychology*, New York: Plenum Press.

Reed, D. L. (1987) 'An empirical phenomenological approach to dream research', in Van Zuuren, F., Wertz, F. J. and Mook, B., eds, *Advances in Qualitative Psychology*, Berwyn, PA: Swets & Zeitlinger.

Rickman, H. P., ed., (1976) *Dilthey: Selected Writings*, Cambridge: Cambridge University Press.

Rose D. (2001) *Users' Voices: The Perspectives of Health Service Users*, London: The Sainsbury Centre for Mental Health.

Todres, L. (1998) 'The qualitative description of human experience: The aesthetic dimension', *Qualitative Health Research*, 8, 1: 121–7.

Todres, L. (1999) 'The bodily complexity of truth-telling in qualitative research: Some implication of Gendlin's philosophy', *Humanistic Psychologist*, 23, 3: 283–300.

Todres, L. (2000) 'Writing phenomenological–psychological descriptions: An illustration attempting to balance texture and structure'. *Auto/Biography*, 3, 1 and 2: 41–8.

Todres, L. (2004) 'The meaning of understanding and the open body: Some implications for qualitative research', *Existential Analysis*, 15, 1: 38–55.

Turner, R., ed., (1974) *Studies in Ethnomethodology*, Harmondsworth: Penguin.

Van Kaam, A. (1959) 'Phenomenal analysis: Exemplified by a study of the experience of really feeling understood', *Journal of Individual Psychology*, 15: 66–72.

Von Eckartsberg, R. (1998) 'Existential–phenomenological research', in Valle, R., ed., *Phenomenological Inquiry in Psychology: Existential and Transpersonal Dimensions*, New York: Plenum Press.

Wertz, F. J. (1983) 'From everyday to psychological description: Analyzing the moments of a qualitative data analysis', *Journal of Phenomenological Psychology*, 14, 2: 197–241.

Wilcock, P. M., Brown, G. C. S., Bateson, J., Carver, J. and Machin, S. (2003) 'Using patient stories to inspire quality improvement within the modernisation agency collaborative programmes', *Journal of Clinical Nursing*, 12: 1–9.

Chapter 5

From the porter's point of view

Participant observation by the interpretive anthropologist in the hospital

Nigel Rapport

Anthropology and interpretation: two incidents

One of the tasks I am often allocated as a porter in Constance Hospital – a large National Health Service teaching and general medical facility in Easterneuk, Scotland – is collecting specimens. As 'specimens-man', on 'the spec-ies run', it is my job, four times a day, to traverse the 30-odd miles of hospital corridor and collect from some 50 wards the blood, urine and cellular samples to go to the biochemistry or microbiology laboratories for analysis. Once I have mapped out the optimal route across the plant linking the different pick-up sites, each run takes me about 80 minutes; but I still find it tedious and lonely, and it leaves me footsore.

One day, between runs, one of the portering charge-hands somewhat sheepishly sends me back to a ward I have only recently visited to pick up an urgent specimen: these cannot await the scheduled pick-ups and are taken for analysis immediately. Arriving in the Ward 7 sluice room I look for an *Urgent* sticker on the couple of specimens I can see hanging on the hook, but I can find none. I ask at the nurses' station. 'Who ordered the porter?', a nurse calls out for me. A young, male student doctor replies that he did, and that he left them on the hook – and he enters the sluice room to show me. 'They're gone!' 'I've got these,' I say, holding up the two in my hand, 'but they're not marked urgent.' 'Oh, sorry,' he says, 'I thought the urgent ones went down the chute and that I was to phone for any others; that's what happened in Ward 9.' I inform him of the correct procedure and stare at him with annoyance. I am pleased when we are now joined in the sluice room by a senior nurse who repeats what I have just said; I keep staring at the junior doctor as he blushes with embarrassment. I am surprised at how much pleasure it gives me.

Whenever the student doctor and I pass in the corridor thereafter we exchange looks. The little grin playing on his lips tells me that he recognises how tiny is my victory in terms of the long-term disparities in what he supposes to be our likely job trajectories and status. ('Have a coffee' is the throwaway line he offers me, magnanimously, some months later, when I have again been called to the ward unnecessarily.)

I am sitting on Mrs Gilbert's bed, beside the wheelchair I have brought up from the front door, waiting for the doctor to sign her out so that I can convey her to the waiting ambulance. We chat about this and that: books, newspapers, politics, her children working down south, her garden. Every now and then a nurse comes over to apologise to her for the delay. Finally the doctor is sighted, comes over to her bed, writes her prescription, and tells her to get a blood test to check the level of Warfarin necessary for her. As he writes and talks rapidly, he leans right across me, as if I'm not there. I find his physical closeness embarrassing and lean back as far as I can: he does not appear to notice.

My work as a porter is not a permanent occupation: I am an anthropologist and university employee conducting research at Constance Hospital on the issue of national identity by way of a year's participant observation.[1] Am I justified in contending that my own reactions to hierarchical relations in the hospital might offer insight into those of the other porters (some 135 men and two women) who are my work-mates? What is the nature of the data I derive from my experience?

Qualitative as against quantitative methodology

A range of methods are employed in modern-day 'sociocultural anthropology'[2] in the gathering of data: conducting interviews, focus group discussions, video-recording, network analysis, transcribing genealogies, censuses, archives, life histories, questionnaires and participant observation. A questioning of the nature of anthropology's methodology pertains to all, however, and speaks to broader issues to do with the nature of the discipline as such – art or science? – regarding, indeed, the nature of scientific knowledge of the human condition – qualitative or quantitative, phenomenological or positivist? The approach adopted in the present chapter will be largely qualitative, phenomenological, 'interpretive'.[3] I treat the interpretive understandings that an anthropologist might deduce from participant observation fieldwork: from 'immersion' in the life-worlds – the everyday words, behaviours, interactions – of other people which has represented the major anthropological method since the early twentieth century.[4]

At the core of the differentiation between so-called qualitative and quantitative approaches in social science is a disagreement over the relationship between knowledge and the replication of information. For something to be true in human life, does it have to be observably replicated or replicatable (quantitative); and does a sample of events of the same kind have to be taken into account so that the representativeness of the new information can be ascertained? Alternatively, can one accept something is true if observed only by one person on one occasion (qualitative), both the manner of observation and the nature of the thing observed precluding replication? Indeed, can something be imagined to be true if it is unique, its own kind, and while implicated in other things is not them and not like them?

Secondary oppositions then follow in the wake of this question of replication, and deepen the division. For instance: is it necessary to explain subjects from an independent, extraneous, purportedly objective standpoint (quantitative), or can explanation be subjective, and admit a particular point of view (qualitative)? Should researchers begin with a directing hypothesis (quantitative), or with an open mind, cleared as far as possible of preconceptions concerning the nature of their research subjects (qualitative)? Should research identify variables and causal relations which, it is hoped, possess universal provenance (quantitative), or is it sufficient to disinter substantive concepts and theories which are known to be locally grounded (qualitative)? Should researchers restrict themselves to sensory observation and the control of reason (quantitative), or allow themselves to empathise, introspect and intuit meanings and relations (qualitative)?

In part, the opposition between the qualitative and the quantitative can be regarded as an anachronism: a throwback to nineteenth-century conceptions of science, and attempts by social science to ape the reputed certainty of its methods of measurement and so borrow from its legitimacy and status. With the advent of twentieth-century science – Einsteinian relativity, quantum mechanics, chaos theory – came a new ethos, however: an appreciation of the contingency, situatedness and intrusiveness – alternatively, the creativeness – of the research process as such. Conveniently summed up by Heisenberg's 'uncertainty principle', here was a realisation that observers are inevitably and inexorably a part of what they observe, so that what researchers confront is 'reality' as apprehended through their own particular prism of perception, and what they gather as results are artefacts of the process of their observation. The research process is an interactive one, and researchers, observers, are at one and the same time interactants: part of the field of events under observation. Any interpretation of the information accrued, therefore, must somehow come to terms with the fact that far from being 'things-in-themselves', true for all places and all times, data are epiphenomena of their means of acquisition and their framework of representation. If there is no 'immaculate perception', and there are 'no facts, only interpretations', as adumbrated by Nietzsche on the cusp of the twentieth century ([1873] 1911), then research observations, interpretations and generalisations are not so readily distinguishable from beliefs, hypotheses and evaluations.

If there is a growing recognition in the natural sciences that 'proofs' are learnt and respected practices common to a paradigm, and 'truth' is 'primarily a matter of fit: fit to what is referred to in one way or another, or to other renderings, or to modes and manners of organisation' (Goodman 1978: 138), then sociocultural anthropology has also come to accept that 'ethnographic reality is actively constructed, not to say invented' (Dumont 1978: 66). To write an authentic anthropological text is less to represent an absolute reality than to fabricate a fit of a particular generic kind between two types of conventional activity (exchanging spoken words and arranging written words), and hence to 'write' social reality. The 'truth' of anthropological accounts, in a celebrated formulation by Roy Wagner, is that anthropologists invent a culture for their informants: here is 'what they imagine to be a plausible explanation of what they understand them generally to have been doing' (1977: 500–1).

This conclusion is disputed, nonetheless, and much anthropological debate continues to occur over the nature of research processes, of research results and of the presenting and appreciating of information. As what should anthropology represent itself if not a 'generalising science' (Ingold 1997)? Surely it is more than merely 'a collection of travellers' tales' (Louch 1966: 160)? For some, however, this ambiguity and uncertainty is all grist to the anthropological mill. Anthropology – 'the most humanistic of the social sciences, the most scientific of the humanities', in a popular designation – has never been comfortably placed within certain categories of disciplinary knowledge, and, indeed, has seen its project as the exploration, and the calling-into-question, of conventional and disciplinary divisions as such. Sociocultural anthropology was 'born omniform', Clifford Geertz has asserted (1983: 21), and should refuse to be bound or restricted by the preconceptions of categorial knowledge. In seeking as complex an appreciation of experience as possible, an appreciation of the ambiguities concerning the nature of knowledge and truth per se should only make anthropology 'more like itself' (cf. Rapport 1997a).

This certainly became Sir Edmund Leach's anthropological message. Drawing inspiration from the eighteenth-century philosopher–scientist Giambattista Vico, Leach set great store by the facility of an anthropologist's 'artistic imagination' (1982: 53). For Vico, the human imagination was to be regarded as a primary tool in a 'new science' which sought to understand the real as opposed to the outwardly observable nature of a human engagement with its environment. Such real knowledge called for an attempted entering into the minds of other people, so that one came to know not only *that* (Caesar was dead) or *how* (to ride a bike) but *what it was like* (to be poor, to be in love, to belong to a community, to be a porter named Jim). Moreover, it was in the nature of this imaginative knowing, or *fantasia*, that it was not analysable except in terms of itself, and it could not be identified except by individual expressions or instantiations.

A conversation

What follows represents an extended case study into the possibility of anthropologists intuiting what it might be like to 'enter into the minds of other people': practising a Vico-esque human science which brings together the experience and imagination of analysts with interpretings of aspects of the lives of others – *others'* experience and imagination – which might reside beneath the surface of observable behaviours.

As an opening instantiation, I find an extract from the following conversation instructive regarding the way in which my own reactions as an anthropological fieldworker-cum-porter at Constance NHS Hospital, Easterneuk, might offer insight into the reactions of my fellow full-time porters. The exchange finds Jim, an experienced porter, and me in the Accident and Emergency ('A and E') porters' lodge; it is his regular or 'dedicated' (in the terminology of the hospital) worksite, and tonight I am helping him out, covering for his normal partner on holiday leave:[5]

JIM: I'm not a crabbed old man or hard to get on with, but I know the procedures, Nigel, and I'll stand by them. (...) I remember walking through Ward 29 with specimens, once, and this doctor says to me, 'Here, take these too.' And I stop, and I'm just in the process of saying 'Fine, but you'll have to phone the front door first, to check someone isn't already coming down for them.' And before I can get the words half out the doctor says: 'Oh! I'll take them myself!'...You know, this is the only place I've worked where there's been a class system! Never worked anywhere like it, Nigel. The porters are at the bottom: they're nothing, rubbish. Or that's how the doctors and nurses think of them. Those at the top are OK. But it's like any class system: the middle classes wanna be like the upper classes, and tread on the working classes, and look down on them, so as to get up themselves. The nurses also wanna get up and be like doctors. No other place I've worked has been like this. Like, you hear the nurses say: 'Oh, such-and-such doctor is on today in A and E – 'Dave''; and they simper up to him, and you think: 'Why are you doing that? Act better than that.' And I hate groups of student doctors standing together, too: treating you like dirt. (...)

NIGEL: Sounds familiar. Is it any better down here? I would have thought it was.

JIM: Well, at nights here, there definitely is a feeling of camaraderie, but I stay in my buckie [lodge]. I know all the nurses and the doctors – and I like them, and get on with most of them – but I still want to stay in here. They give me cakes, and pavlova, and things ...

NIGEL: That's nice ...

JIM: Yes, it is, but I usually say, 'No'.

NIGEL: Cos it's like, charity.

JIM: Yes, it's too much like charity. And you know that however nice they've been, as soon as there's an alert they will come in here and say: 'Porter? Now!' ... A kind of line will come down [Jim draws a hand down before his face], a fence. And you know all this 'Jim this' and 'Jim that' before had not been real. That's why I wouldn't feel comfortable joining them in the dining room – and they have invited me – 'cos I'd know

that some there would be thinking: 'What's a porter doing in here?' ...
The chief consultant here, McIlvray, is a young man. Forty. Maybe less.
And he still walks past me without noticing me or recognising he knows
me; and I've worked here since A and E opened. I mean, some of the
other consultants are OK, but still ...

What I intend is an elaboration and analysis of a number of the themes the
above conversation turns on: hierarchy, distance, class, discrimination, con-
testation. This case study in interpretive anthropology will thus take the form
of a combination of my own experiences as a porter at Constance Hospital,
my record of interactions with other porters, and my construing of porters'
experiences, as evidenced in these interactions, in the light of my own.

Hierarchy and its obviation: eight propositions

I offer now eight analytical propositions concerning the complex of porters'
relations and attitudes to doctors in Constance Hospital, by which I would
summarise the porter's point of view: an experience of hospital hierarchy,
and its obviation.

1. Being a porter means coming to terms with being a nothing, at the base of a hospital hierarchy topped by doctors

The coercive nature of the institution of the hospital became apparent to me
on the morning of my formal induction into the job of portering. For more
than an hour, Pat, the portering sub-manager, dinned into me and six other
neophytes a list of rules (regarding timekeeping, cleanliness, smoking, uni-
form and dress, telephone etiquette, patient-handling, safety and
confidentiality), as well as the punishments for their infraction. At the same
time the institution's hierarchical nature was made plain. 'You might think
porters are a small cog in a large machine,' Pat remarked, 'but don't think
you're nothing just because people say you are. People might say you're
"just a porter" but it's not true; no part of the hospital could run without
you – the same with domestics.' *Being a porter meant dealing with being a
nothing.* This was a notion I was to find regularly repeated – as it was by
Jim, above ('The porters are at the bottom: they're nothing, rubbish. Or
that's how the doctors and nurses think of them.').

The low status of the porter, and the diametric contrast with that of the
doctor, was signalled and made manifest in a number of ways: *in our uni-
form or dress* (for the porter, blue or yellow polo shirt with name badge and
title – 'Support Services' – irrevocably ironed on, and blue canvas trousers;
for the doctor, civilian dress and tie, with removable name-badge, possibly
with white coat, or else operating-theatre greens); *in the different manner in
which we were addressed* (or ignored); *in the different parts of the hospital*

plant our statuses led us to occupy, and the ways we would traverse the plant in fulfilment of our duties; *in our differential knowledge of the running of the institution* and the input we had into its policy; in our pay and our possibilities for advancement; *in the homes and holidays we went to outside the institution*, and the modes of transport that took us there.

I was soon introduced to what the distance between porters and doctors meant in practice. Roger, one of the porters who began with me, confessed, with some shame, that he'd been told off that morning: he'd kept a doctor waiting in the operating theatre because a patient he was sent to collect was not ready in the ward, and he hadn't remembered to phone in to explain that the delay was not his fault. Not long after, I found myself challenged: a senior nurse ordered me peremptorily into a doctors' ward-room to explain why I had mistakenly taken a particular patient to X-ray. Fortunately I could give an account of the instructions I received via my bleeper and a woman in the room corroborated my story and apologised: it was her error. After I was ushered out of the room again the senior nurse turned to me, impressed: 'There! You just had an apology from the head doctor on the ward! A senior registrar! I said to them: "That porter's stressed! And I keep getting his name wrong [she laughed], and calling him Angel!" It's cos *Angel* is on TV tonight. Do you watch that?' Not only, I was to understand, did a doctor's apology more than compensate for a mistaken interrogation, but the thought of a stressed porter was somewhat amusing; meanwhile, it was friendliness to talk down to my level by way of soap operas that removed us both from the hospital context.

I learnt, then, that porters are not to be taken so seriously. Not only are we not to be particularly trusted in the carrying out of our duties, but those duties themselves, the regulations surrounding them, and the time it takes us to fulfil them are not particularly valued. On one occasion I found myself with two portering managers keeping fire doors closed in a corridor as alarms blared and firemen rushed into an operating theatre and then down to the kitchens; the fact it was another false alarm did not cancel out the ignominy as doctors ostentatiously ignored the alarm, the regulations and us, and walked, casually chatting, through the fire doors and to their destinations without breaking stride. Peggy Cox, my manager, held up her hands to me through the glass door-panel in exasperation – embarrassed, also, that I had witnessed her irrelevancy.

At the core of my initial reaction to being a porter around doctors – a 'nothing' at the base of a hospital hierarchy – was a sense of indignity and of shame. And I was heartened that my fellow neophyte, Roger, seemed to feel this too:

ROGER: I had a busy morning, Nigel. [He puts on a loud English-sounding voice.] 'Do this. Return with this. Do that …' 'Nae bother' … But you know, it's not right what I'm made to do in the theatres. Like clean the doctors' clogs after the operations! I mean, who knows what's on them after an operation ...The doctors just leave them, and their greens, on the floor and I have to go in and clear up. And clean the floors.

NIGEL: Don't the domestics do that?

ROGER: The domestics come in after. But I'm a porter! Why should I do that? I'm gonna write a letter of complaint ... I was told that porters do the job cos they always have. But that's not right. That's just porters not having the guts to stand up and say 'No'. I'm only wearing little rubber gloves, and my greens. I could catch anything. And I'm not properly trained for the job either; I haven't been told what to do and what to avoid, like.'

The fact that Roger and I were neophytes is significant, as we shall see. But it is also noteworthy how soon after his arrival in the job Roger's statement that he was 'A porter!' came to carry with it a sense of independence, also of righteousness; he had rights as well as duties, he had the ability to remain civil and retain a sense of proportion ('Nae bother'), and he had the means and the confidence to seek redress. But not just yet. The first proposition to learn with regard to being a porter, I would suggest, is that one's time, one's work, one's happiness, health and comfort count for very little in an hierarchical order of things topped by the routines of the doctors.

2. Being a porter means being ignorant about what life for the doctors at the top of the hospital hierarchy actually entails, and vice versa

Independent of considerations of status, the hospital as an administered unit is based on a differentiation of knowledge, skills and working practices across the plant. In a sense, this differentiation is functional to the hospital's running and efficiency. The porters and doctors do not need to know the same things; if they did know, it might in fact jeopardise the optimal fulfilment of their duties – knowing how to doctor might be an irrelevancy in terms of the skills and practices over which the porter has to maintain competency, not to mention the sense of frustration that might accrue due to having skills that cannot be operationalised. It is also the case that the division of labour and the mutual ignorance this engenders facilitates the administration of the institution: the administrators' task is made easier if they control information that divides their staff; while training expensively – medically – only those staff who need particular (high-status) skills in doctoring is cheaper than training all to the same level.

Besides the knowledge that their ignorance of the life of doctoring translates into a lack of status, however, the porters find this ignorance also to be a source of anxiety. For, in order to be guaranteed the ability to carry out their portering duties, porters must assure themselves of some knowledge of doctors' practice – their use of space and time, the meaning of their commands, the extent of their power to lessen or increase the portering load, the implications of failing them – and there is a worry that this knowledge may not be acquired. There was a sense in which I found the porters regarding it as part of their duty to find out for themselves the knowledge necessary to fulfil their duties; it had to be by their own efforts because no one else could be relied upon.

Working in the mail room was not a popular location among the porters' own internal rankings, partly because of the tedium: a small group of staff – without, therefore, much chance for relief – sorting through some 7,000 letters per day (not including parcels), franking some 3,500 items of outgoing mail, and delivering three times a day along three different routes around the hospital. The level of knowledge of particular doctors' names and locations which this required – not to mention that of student doctors who did not stay put for any length of time – meant that the room for error, and for being seen to have made a mistake, was large, and more than in other kinds of engagement with doctors. Porters' anxiety, indeed, might be said to be attached to each item of delivered mail – making that anxiety all the more tangible and identifiable (and the job unpopular).

3. Being a porter means turning the distance and ignorance between porters and doctors into a source of stereotypical and apocryphal otherness

The ignorance of the porters regarding doctors, the distance between the bottom of the hospital hierarchy and the top, represents a kind of informational vacuum or black hole. One way in which the porters resist being swallowed up by their ignorance – being drawn into anxiety as a workaday condition – is to fill the vacuum with their own apocrypha or mythology concerning doctors; from black hole to black box, if you will, in which all manner of stereotypical data are stored, compassing doctors' otherness. Doctors' practices, their characters, habits and failings become the stuff of portering lore, into which neophytes are socialised, and of which all routinely remind themselves as explanatory resources. Mishap, failure, wonder and chaos can be explicated by way of doctor-others whose stereotypical distance from oneself conjures them up as convenient objects of fear, dislike, criticism, laughter, even transcendence.

One never knew what one was carrying in the specimens' supposedly sealed polythene packages, Dugald informed me: 'It could be AIDS, anything,' and 'You can't be too careful.' For while it was the case that particularly virulent specimens ought to bear a red dot, and the doctors ought always to put dotted ones on top of the pile, they sometimes forgot to do either. Porters had to look out for themselves because the doctors were lax. Sometimes specimens got lost, Old John continued; the doctors took them to the laboratories themselves, perhaps, then forget they had done so and tried to put the blame on the porter. Or else the doctors prepared a specimen, then forgot about it and it lay on their desk for a few hours – or days; then they remembered and the specimen showed up on the hook in the sluice room with a time or a date long passed – with the porter then getting accused of not doing his rounds. The point is to know what doctors might get up to and to stand your ground if cheeked.

Being uncaring and devious was not the end of the characteristics I was led to expect from doctors, moreover. 'Dr Doolittle' was a lighthearted moniker the porters would appropriate to signal doctors' nonchalant laziness, but this critique could also give rise to more serious revelations. For doctors' laziness translated into incapacity:

JIM: The whole place is dirty, Nigel, filthy. All the cross infection...And what do they expect? They get porters cleaning the Main Theatres – someone like Roger who does not want or like the job and does not do it properly. All the clogs get thrown into the domestics' sink – just to the left when you enter Main Theatre – and they're meant to be disinfected. But Roger says he just washes them. Then the cleaners use that sink to get water to clean all the surfaces...Those clogs will have dried blood caked on them. Cos the Theatre floors get filthy with blood, you know; and blood really does travel. Really, all the walls and roof should be cleaned. I know doctors only claim to be sterile from the waist up, but still...

Also, doctors worked in an arcane and non-rational fashion:

STEVE: Do you know what day it is today?
NIGEL: Wednesday?
STEVE: Its 'Cock-up City'! The day all the doctors change wards – and all want X-rays. [I look nonplussed.] Every six months, Nigel, all the student doctors change wards – change their specialities, like – so that they can move up from Junior to Senior House Officers. And as soon as they get to a new ward they say: 'Right: I want everyone X-rayed or scanned; I don't care how recently it's been done before!'

Doctors were also socially inept:

MARTIN: Most people who work here are OK. But the doctors are arrogant: think they're better than the rest. And they're ignorant too; even when they used to see me with my mail trolley they'd not move out of way. They have no discretion, no social skills, at all.

Lastly, there is an appreciation that the stereotypical and apocryphal way in which porters construe doctors will be reciprocated, since the distance and ignorance that divides them is mutual. When Fred hears it is my last day as a porter, and that next I begin engaging with the doctors, he warns me with a laugh: 'They'll be giving you dog's abuse about the porters, Nigel, you know that, don't you? They'll be telling you how they're a load of shite. And they'll be right, of course! At least about some of them! Won't they?'

4. Being a porter means turning the distance and ignorance between doctors and porters into a kind of contractual stand-off

Transforming their ignorance of doctors into characterisations of an apocryphal and stereotypical – a known and expectable, even if regrettable – kind delivers a note of bullishness to porters' voices. Porters can successfully look out for themselves; porters can see doctors for what they are; porters can give as good as they get; porters can see the funny sides of the demeaning situations in which the hierarchicalisation of the hospital places them. The logic of this bullishness, ironically enough, can be explained in terms of the hospital hierarchy, now flattened into a division of labour in which each part supplies something the others lack: by virtue of the division of labour each kind of worker has a power base – of skills, routines and peers – to call their own. It matters less that some suppliers engage in demeaning labour (or that others seem to disrespect that labour and the skills behind it) than that by the terms of the institution the right to supply that (demeaning) labour is vested in some workers alone. A contractual relationship of differential supply and demand, in short, regulates the interaction of porters and doctors; the distance between them means that porters can feel their labour is needed, and that they have a right to redress if the proprieties of that distance are not maintained.

It was a common refrain in the porters' lodge that doctors would be lost without porters' physical prowess and skills. On one occasion, Steve returned from the wards with news of a 'loony patient still refusing treatment'; this then reminded him of other instances of a patient 'going mental':

STEVE: Gary McMurdo [a porter] got the plaudits for knocking out a guy in Ward 5, remember? All the doctors were sitting round not knowing what to do, as this patient went mad with a needle, rushing round stabbing things. Like IV bags. So, Gary says to me: 'Here, hold these curtains closed!', then he goes in and deals with the patient! And after that the patient didn't leave his bed the whole of the day! [He laughs.]

Not only do porters know that their physical prowess marks them off in the hospital and assures them of a skill and a place that no one else can gainsay or approach, they also display confidence in this physicality as a route to redress when their institutional rights are threatened. They might threaten to withdraw their physical labour – take industrial action and walk out on strike – or they might turn their physical power against the institution, against the doctors, as such. When Wilbur quizzed me, then, about delivering an urgent specimen from Ward 31 because a doctor had been on the phone claiming the laboratory never received it, Henry (overhearing) advised me to 'do as Phil once did: go down there and hit the doctor about!' Henry was only half-joking, but Wilbur murmured his agreement.

Meanwhile I took it as a sign of Roger's continuing passage from neophyte to established hand when one day he confessed to me:

ROGER: I'm gonna start telling people straight, what I think of them. Sod it! ... You know, Roy McMadden nearly hit a doctor yesterday! 'Come on then! If you want it, come on then!' he said. Aye!

NIGEL: Why?!

ROGER: Oh, the doctor had been moaning at him all day, like...In the end the doctor sent him an apology but Roy had had enough by then and was going home. But he said if he sees him again today he's gonna shove a catheter up his arse!

5. Being a porter means having the potential to develop the contractual stand-off with doctors into relations of a joking and casual kind

We have seen that by virtue of the institutional division of labour in the hospital, and the mutual ignorance between the top of the hierarchy and the bottom, porters feel themselves to possess a certain contractual security – a place in the institution and a set of skills that are by rights theirs alone. They play on this security, moreover, to engender a sense of portering pride, righteousness and, if necessary, bloody-mindedness.

It is also the case, however, that as an occupational group, even a community (with members, traditions and lore), porters can now look beyond themselves to the group of doctors with some confidence, even magnanimity, and construe a range of possible and growing relations between 'us' and 'them'. Once porters are assured of who they are – are institutionally confirmed as being – then possibilities exist regarding how others, outsiders, might relate to them and know them. Porters and doctors become two group entities linked by a diversity of possible kinds and moments of their coming together: in love and war, in play and seriousness.

This can even extend to kinds of relations that replace and transcend the very institutional relations that caused the identification, the separation and the possible coming together, of 'us' and 'them', in the first place. The hospital division of labour transmogrifies into a field of social possibilities that ranges beyond the logic of the institution as such. Deriving a confidence from membership of a social–occupational community empowers the porters to engage with doctors in ways which joke about, make light of, diverge from, even obviate, the very statuses of 'porters' and 'doctors' and the institutional ignorance and distance of which these statuses are constituted.

It is often sufficient for porters merely to introduce relations they have outside the hospital into their relations with doctors for their (hierarchical) statuses inside the hospital to be transformed. This was the case when Jim explained to me how he 'inherited' a contraband business, selling cut-price cigarettes and such like round the hospital, from a porter who was just leaving. Jim followed in the latter's footsteps, selling all over the hospital – and to everyone, doctors and nurses included. He stopped when he became a dedicated Accident and Emergency porter (and did not get to move around so much) but till then he had as many cigarettes for himself as he liked, and the doctors 'used to come to him and queue up'!

It is the case, indeed, that the relations with the outside world that the porters introduce into the hospital domain (to effect a transcending of porter–doctor differentiations) can be as ephemeral and immaterial as a matter of reputation – the porters' confidence in their sex appeal, for instance. One morning, then, Dwayne ran into me in Ward 36 where he was awaiting a patient:

DWAYNE: Do you ever chat up the doctors, Nigel?
NIGEL: Chat them up! Doctors don't even look at you! [Dwayne walks over to two young female doctors standing at the nurses' station, has a few quiet words with them and soon both turn towards me, grin, and say theatrically: 'Hello, Nigel.' Next, Dwayne puts his arm round the waist of one of them and leads her over to me.]
DWAYNE: This is Sarah. [She smiles, I blush.] I've been chatting her up for years!
SARAH: I'm sorry I've never said 'Hello' to you before, Nigel, but from now on I will. Whenever I see you pass by.

I explain they are embarrassing me and they stop. Dwayne retrieves his patient, and as he pushes the bed away with an accompanying nurse I hear him assure her that she does not 'have to bend over and help him push' because then he'll 'have to be looking at her fat bum'.

Whenever Dwayne and I meet thereafter he informs me of his latest conquests – he's chatted to another doctor, 'a little blonde one in Ward 19, Nora Jane' – and he announces to other porters how much happier I am now that doctors are talking to me.

6. Being a porter means being used to regarding doctors as authority figures in everyday life, and bringing this regard into the hospital as a means to domesticate the work environment

It is of course the case that 'porters' and 'doctors' inside the institution of the hospital replay the relations that exist between 'patients' and 'doctors' in everyday life. 'Doctors' are not an unknown quantity to porters, or role-players that exist only within the working environment of the hospital; and knowing doctors in the everyday world, having personal relations with a doctor – 'their' doctor – in the wider context of their lives, can be expected to impinge upon how the porters relate to doctors in the work context of the hospital.

In part, this is a relationship of inequality that carries over into the work-place. However, coming to regard the distance and ignorance that separates them from doctors in the hospital hierarchy as a continuation of their every-day lives can also be used by porters to more paradoxical effect: to soften or domesticate this status differential and the feelings of worthlessness that might accompany it. For 'everyday life' comprises a complex array of feel-ings and statuses, and by reminding oneself that one's distance from one's doctor in everyday life is but a small part of that life – its contests, victories and defeats – one can reappraise, recontextualise, the distancing effect of the workplace, and likewise see in it the existence of a diversity of sources and kinds of self-esteem.

I take this bringing of a home relationship with the medical profession into the context of the workplace to be one reason too for the extent to which the porters gossip about their own ill-health and ailments to one another; being sick and being at work – both involving face-to-face rela-tions with doctors – are similar, temporary conditions which they might expect to overcome.

The very first day I met my fellow-neophyte, Roger, he informed me that he was a premature baby, that he had recently had a hernia operation to clear a testicular swelling the size of a tennis ball, and that his dyslexia meant he suffered from poor coordination. ('Say you asked me to touch my right hand to my left ear, I could do it about 50 per cent of the time. (...) My parents were always very good about it – they brought me up great – but they didn't know why my coordination was bad; then a doctor told them it was also part of my dyslexia.') How he overcame his coordi-nation problems through karate training was to become part of Roger's and my daily fare. Similarly, the very high arches with which Luke was born ('My mum told me I couldn't walk till I was three, and that's why I still bounce when I walk now') are regularly introduced into conversation in order to explain why he must refrain from five-a-side football with the other porters:

> The doctor said I should cut out football now that I'm ageing. I just had two Cortisone injections in my heels – they've grown spurs – but my high arches will need built-up shoes to support them. The doctor said the injections will help a bit, but in the end what I need is an operation.

Routine talk of their bodily complaints, signing themselves into Accident and Emergency when they felt unwell, did not seem to detract from the porters' sense of their manliness. In part, I think, this was a matter of getting the care that was due to them: getting the free medical attention that was their right and that the high-status medical profession (whose workings were so blatant a part of their workaday milieu) was funded to provide. But the point is also, I feel, that everyone made trips to the doctor's – Constance was full of the sick – and most people walked out of the surgery at the end of the consultation. Most people, in other words, recovered from their interaction with doctors; the porters, too, might expect to live healthily beyond the unequal exchanges that characterised their workaday routines.

It was also the case that the authority of doctors in everyday life could be brought to bear upon the institution of the hospital in a more direct way, so as to effect an immediate release of the porters from its strictures and control. 'Tame' doctors – doctors who were part of one's domestic world – could sign porters off work while still making them eligible for sick-pay. There was a recognised route to being on sick-leave (as we have seen), even for a number of weeks consecutively, and porters were confident in their ability to traverse it without hindrance; it was part of their contractual security. One sustained an injury – in sport, say, or in a pub fight – one produced a doctor's note and one got one's shop steward to ratify an 'insurance line'. Worrying over the niceties of one's cover was something the union officials and also the portering charge-hands regarded as part of their pastoral management roles, and I was struck by how certain and relaxed the porters would seem in effecting the proprieties.

In the same way that porters can rely on their rights to assure themselves of a division of labour in their relations with doctors *inside* the hospital, so they are assured of certain rules in their working conditions which enable them to use their relations with doctors *outside* the hospital to exert pressure on their working institution.

7. Being a porter means using knowledge of everyday life to lessen the import of the hospital hierarchy and the authority of doctors as such

I have argued that bringing their home relationships with doctors into the context of the hospital is a symbolic means which porters use to soften or domesticate the status differentials they find at work and their feelings of worthlessness. More than this, however, the link to home, the wider world and everyday life can become a route to a perceived equality, even transcendence. The hospital, porters recognise, is not the only space – is not the normal or modal or paradigmatic space for the world at large – and doctors, their provenance, knowledge, skills and relevance, diminish in power in the context of everyday practices – popularities and potentialities, excesses and novelties – which they do not control, of which they might be wholly ignorant. Outside the hospital, in the world at large, doctors may be simply human beings; doubly diminished, indeed, by the distances they fall from their workaday affectations.

Part of the stereotypical condition under which porters lived in the hospital was that, in character, they were all 'chirpy, cheeky chappies', as Steve, a Londoner, phrased it for me. That is, the doctors, nurses, administrators and patients alike saw them, at least in part, as clownish figures: a source of light relief in a generally stricken milieu. Porters served both as the butt of others' humour and as tricksters who embodied a Peter Pan-ish world where responsibility, seriousness and skill were not issues. Sometimes porters would act out cameos of these stereotypes for the amusement of doctors and patients, and themselves. More often, however, they turned their supposed trickster connections with an easy-going outside world on the inmates of the institution themselves – and on the doctors in particular.

Thus it was, for instance, that doctors became mere objects of porters' sexual appetites:

MARTIN: Some beautiful women in the hospital, eh Nige [as we pass a young doctor]? And with see-through uniforms – just to make the time better for the porters, like, as they pass by! [We laugh.]

DWAYNE: [staring at a young female doctor] The things you see when you don't have an erection! [He screws his face up in mock yearning.]

It is also the case that doctors-as-objects possess despicable personal habits, and can thus be seen actually as responsible for diminishing themselves. In clearing out a doctor's rest-room prior to a ward refurbishment, therefore, Dugald and I picked gingerly through the personal possessions before he advised me simply to 'bin everything': 'Doctors are filthy, pigs, in their personal habits.'

The point of this objectification is not now to delineate a stereotypical and apocryphal other, with whom one is bound to engage in working relations within the hospital division of labour, but to call the very judgements behind that division into question. One is insisting on seeing the individuals behind the role-players, and drawing attention to personal qualities and inadequacies which unfit doctors for their roles, which call into the question the very status of 'doctor' as such.

This was clear in the relish with which porters would rehearse accounts of medical mistakes for which doctors had been responsible. Roger's testicular hernia was, it transpires, first misdiagnosed as a varicose vein and operated upon. Only when the pain drove Roger back to the hospital did they admit it was lucky he returned when he did, because his stomach wall had just split.

Not only is it the case that doctors are unfit for their own jobs (and status) but also that in many cases the porters possess more medical expertise in diagnosing and curing. Thus it is that Bob recounted how he 'eventually got [his] way' with a doctor unwilling to provide him with a steroid injection for his knee. The doctor argued that the little muscle content in that part of the body could mean dangerous consequences, but Bob, as a body-builder, knew better how fast he could 'put on muscle'.

This adds up to a sense not only that doctors are fakes in the claims they make, the airs they assume, the status they are accorded, but also that they are fools. They take themselves too seriously, take their work too seriously, put too much store by their supposed skills, the hospital, its hierarchies and institutional regime. They miss out on the fun that life is really about.

This is something that Roger, my fellow-neophyte (and keen rock-band member), came to appreciate after a number of months in the job:

ROGER: Anne [the portering manager] said to me that my job here was the real thing and should be more important to me than my band!... What!? Is she kidding? Has she never had FUN? These people round here never have fun...You know, only the porters round here have a sense of humour. Like, I was messing round outside the theatre the other day [he grins in remembrance], me and Roy McMadden, just having a bit of fun about putting paper in bins, and this guy comes out of the theatre and says: 'This is an Operating Theatre!' [he puts on a serious, officious, more English-sounding voice]. Probably a doctor: they act like they're automatons. 'Do this, do that', they tell you, just like you're one too.

Meanwhile, the way that Roger succeeds in turning the area outside the operating theatre where he is stationed into what Wilbur describes fondly as a kind of 'heavy-metal disco' – Roger playing 'air guitar' and 'blam-blamming' in time to the rock music emanating from his music system as doctors and patients process by, becomes a proud part of portering lore.

The implication is that doctors, positioned outside the porters' world, are also in a way outside life's real processes and passages; wed to a hospital regimen, doctors fail to apprehend the nitty-gritty of life.

8. Being a porter means recognising doctors as fellow human beings trying, like them, to make do and get on in a world of institutions, rules, norms and circumstances they do not control

One day I see a small photograph taped to a white board near the nurses' station and doctors' desk in Ward 14; it is of the student doctor whom I was pleased to embarrass previously, when he got the specimens' procedure wrong in Ward 7 sluice room. I take a closer look; a drawing around the photograph makes his head seemingly part of a turkey; two intravenous drips enter the turkey's body, while exiting onto the floor is a catheter tube and bag. My emotions towards the doctor are, as ever, mixed, but I cannot help feeling a little sorry for his being publicly teased. Life for the porters, I have suggested, its nitty-gritty wholeness, is generally to be found beyond the hospital institution, and doctors can be seen to miss out on it inasmuch as they are more entangled in the institution, more co-opted into its hierarchy. Porters transcend the hospital and become real and distinguished human actors but doctors do not.

This can, however, also translate into a sense of pity and of sympathy that the porters extend to doctors: an equalitarian ethos that we are all human beings, trying to make do. Porters will emphasise, for instance, how doctors are under the same institutional strictures as they are. If a doctor is on weekend shift, then, as Kevin commiserates with a glum-looking one: 'You'll not be out drinking then!' Meanwhile, a doctor leaving Constance for a new job in Exeter – and for whose leaving party (and pub-crawl) I had seen an invitatory notice pinned to Ward 36 – I was to meet in the house of my St. Andrews neighbour. 'Did I know the porters Rory and Dwayne?' Lance, the doctor, wanted to know.

I mentioned my chance meeting to Dwayne when I next saw him:

DWAYNE: Aye, Rory and me went to his going-away party! How did you meet him?
NIGEL: At my neighbour's; he's a physiotherapist.
DWAYNE: And did this neighbour play rugby?
NIGEL: Yeah!
DWAYNE: That's Lance [laughing]: rugby mad.
NIGEL: How did you meet?
DWAYNE: I met Lance at Easterneuk Royal Infirmary, where he did his four years' training. Then we both moved here. He's been here about seven years, so I've known him about 11. Good bloke! He promised me a job reference if I wanted one – cos you can't trust these [portering] chargehands!

As a friend, Dwayne can expect Lance to help him leave behind Constance Hospital, its divisions and intrigues, as Lance himself has now done. Friends are not compassed by the statuses of 'porter' and 'doctor'.

Discussion

The eight propositions I have outlined above, as a description of the complex of relations and attitudes which the porters of Constance Hospital possess with regard to doctors, have come to take something of a processual form. Beginning with the nothingness of porters in the hospital hierarchy and the mutual ignorance that separates the top of the hierarchy from the base, there is a progression through stereotyping and contractual stand-off, and through joking relations, to a domestication of the institutional hospital space, the diminishment of its import, and lastly the democratic impulse that sees doctors and porters alike as faced with institutional coercion, and able to help one another through. Here is a story of hierarchy and its obviations: of transcending institutional differentiation so as to arrive at relations deriving from an existential, or at least wider, social awareness, and giving onto a generically human community. Victor Turner (1982) famously described this as 'the ritual process': a common human practice of moving experientially from structure and classification in everyday life to a more 'liminal' state (in the margins of that life), where we engage in non-structural, even anti-structural, relations with our fellow human beings, now recognised as facing the same existential conditions; from workaday institutionalism to a sense of universal 'communitas' where true worth and real communion are achieved. Was this at the back of my mind when I framed my eight propositions in processual, progressive or narrative form from institution to transcendence?

In part, I think it was my personal experience which has led me to present porter–doctor relations as I have, an experience which included knowing certain anthropological texts and theories – such as Turner's – and, more nearly, of approaching being a porter from the position of being a professional anthropologist. The hospital institution, its hierarchy, the everyday indignities of being a porter, were all, initially, and suddenly, oppressive to me; I extrapolate from my sense of oppression to my fellows', and have us *all* share the need for transcendence, and so present us as travelling alike an experiential route from hierarchy to its obviation.

But have I the right to make this extrapolation? Inducted into being a 'nothing' at the base of a hierarchy was novel to me, something which did not accord with my sense of self, my self-esteem, or the way I had become used to being esteemed by others; but for my fellow porters at Constance this might have been a constant aspect of their lives. I enter the hospital with the knowledge that 'in another life' it is the doctors who are my natural interlocutors, but my fellow porters do not necessarily own this expectation or feel my shock of non-recognition. I have since stopped – 'escaped' – being a porter, but some of my fellows in Constance have not. I have replaced – 'escaped' – the post-industrial cityscape of Easterneuk for the charms of St. Andrews, but many of my erstwhile fellows in Constance will not.

But, in part, I believe also that the above eight propositions contain a kind of developmental or ontological logic which suggests itself to me as a consequence of my experiential immersion in the hospital as a field-site. I did not see or consciously know the progression contained above until I began to consider writing this analysis (cf. Lambert and McKevitt 2002: 212). It delivered itself up to me as the logical way in which my notes from my fieldwork made sense. (I am heartened to see how my fellow-neophyte porter, Roger, also traversed a relational and attitudinal evolution, then, from the self-mortification of our induction, through a retaliatory bloody-mindedness, to a recognition that a wider world and fuller life still impinged on that of the hospital and contained the roots of the latter's obviation.) In other words, I would claim for the above progression a coming-together of my experience as an anthropological fieldworker, as a part-time volunteer porter at Constance Hospital, with a processual form which characterises interactions between porters and doctors in the hospital, and porters' atti-tudes to these. I would claim to have experienced and recounted something that takes me beyond a life-world that simply reflects my own expectations, relations and attitudes before entering the field, to a symbolic and structural form which characterises social life at Constance. I cannot claim to have become a (full-time) porter; I cannot claim to have entered into the minds of other porters in anything but an intuitive, subjective sense. But I would claim to have accrued the experiences whereby I can make an informed assumption concerning what being another *is like*, through a comparison of my own experiences with interpretings of others' words and behaviours.

What I would also say is that if the above progression from hierarchical induction to obviation encompasses the story of my own fieldwork experi-ence from university to hospital and back to university, then for many of the porters the progression nevertheless represents a continuing part of their life within the hospital institution. Living the logical progression of these eight propositions may not move the porters out of the institution – although there is quite a high turnover rate, with porters coming, going and returning to this job among other (low-paid, unskilled) ones and none – but living the propositions' logical progression is still done mentally and affectively, on a daily basis, *in* the hospital; the progression becomes a cognitive resort, a coping strategy, with which porters deal with the constancy of the hospital's institutionalism.

Finally, I do not want to claim that the above progression represents the only way in which these eight propositions are used by porters in Constance, for the eight also exist independently of one another, in their own right, and might be differently related together. Not all the porters may know or effect all the propositions, and some may occupy one or more rela-tional and attitudinal positions in the hospital – as fearful, say, that their ignorance of doctors may jeopardise their ability properly to fulfil their por-tering duties, or as downplaying the respect due to accorded doctors on account of their personal failings – to the exclusion of all other propositions. Here is a range of attitudes and relations, a bundle of possible traits, and porters will distinguish themselves individually from one another according to whether they treat this range progressively, and unidirectionally, or whether they favour one part of the range over another in terms of the time and importance they accord it. Day to day, moment to moment, even the same porter may treat the propositions differently. They form a logical progression but their narrative may be brought to life, experienced, lived, in a number of ways.

Conclusion: narrative and truth

Since 'the only ego I know at first hand is my own' (1989: 138), Edmund Leach argued for anthropological research to be recognised and accepted as a subjective process whose 'data' represented 'a kind of harmonic projection of the observer's own personality' (1984: 22). Inevitably, each anthropologist saw something which no other would recognise. But this still made the results of anthropological research admissible as knowledge because the aim was not 'objective truth' but 'insight' into behaviour, one's own as well as others': a 'quality of deep understanding' equivalent to 'fully understanding the nuances of a language [as opposed to] simply knowing the dictionary glosses of individual words' (1982: 52). Insight made anthropological writings 'interesting in themselves' – full of meaning, intended and unintended – and not revelatory of 'the external world' so much as of the author's reactions and interactions with it (1984: 22).

In this, Leach comes close to the tenor of suggestions by physics Nobel laureate Igor Prigogine (1989). For Prigogine, an appreciation of the instability and creativity inherent in our world, the impossibility of absolute control or precise forecasting, and a clearer view of the place of human activity-within-the-world, now bring the projects of natural science and social science close to one another. In both, old notions of determinism, materialism and reductionism, of knowledge as omniscient and timeless, must give way to 'a narrative element' in the way we conceive of our knowledge, represent it, and act upon its implications. For, '[i]n effect, all human and social interaction and all literature is the expression of uncertainty about the future, and of a construction of the future' (1989: 389).

An emphasis on narrative, on the implications of their constructions of orderly worlds for the social environments in which human beings live, in turn spurs a treating of social worlds and their representation as 'personal documents'. As a generic category of writing which includes diaries, autobiographies, life histories and letters (cf. Allport 1942), personal documents have long had a respected place in certain, more humanistic versions of social-scientific practice. What is different now, perhaps, is a matter of emphasis and evaluation. There is an appreciation of the 'personal document' of human society and culture not as a partial component, a biased version, an over-determined manifestation, false consciousness or whatever, but *as all there is.*

From qualitative versus quantitative methods of knowledge acquisition, this chapter has progressed to a foregrounding of the narrative nature of our human being-in-the-world, and a coming to terms with knowledge processes which are constructive and interpretational. The growth of an awareness of narrative, and a self-consciousness awareness – anthropology as in itself mediated by the narrational, epistemologically and representa-tionally – has changed radically the perceived nature of the disciplinary endeavour: given it a 'literary turn' (cf. Rapport 1994). As urged by Rodney Needham (1978: 75–6); a 'counsel of perfection' might see anthropologists now reassessing their tasks, their standards, their ambitions, and contem-plating what the discipline might become if it were to break free from its present academicism. Might not anthropology one day achieve something possessing the humane significance of metaphysics and art, Needham won-ders, if ethnographic interpretations were written with the imaginative acuity, the empathetic penetration and the literary artistry of a George Eliot, a Dostoevsky or a Virginia Woolf?

Because of the novelist's command of the personal life of the individual, and because of the novel's wish to connect up what was externally observ-able in a life with what was internally experienced, E. M. Forster (1984) once opined that literature was 'truer' than social science. For, while each person knew from experience that there was much beyond the 'outer' evi-dence of observation, and while social scientists claimed to be equally concerned to record human character, the latter appeared content to restrict themselves to what could be known of its existence from scouring 'the exte-rior surface' of social life only, and to what could approximately be deduced from people's actions, words and gestures. Only the novelist was deter-mined to accrue a fuller knowledge and to seek out 'the hidden life at its [individual] source' (1984: 55–6). Increasingly, however, the distinction Forster would draw no longer suffices. Anthropologists admit that novelists have dealt better than social scientists in the past with 'the subtleties, inflec-tions and varieties of individual consciousness which are concealed by the categorical masks' of membership in social and cultural groups (Cohen 1994: 180). There are, moreover, attempts in growing numbers to remedy the practice. In an anthropology of personal documentation, and an anthro-pology as personal documentation, the impersonalising impulses of an earlier social science are becoming eschewed (cf. Rapport 1997b; Rapport 2002). Here we find the particularities of individual lived experience no longer necessarily eclipsed by generalisation, or otherwise reduced, abstracted, typified or over-determined according to the axioms of a seem-ing-scientific regularity, stability, order or control, but an appreciation of social milieux themselves as complex, personal documents of ongoing, mul-tiple individual construction and interpretation.

Acknowledgements

The research on which this paper reports was funded by the Leverhulme Trust (grant no. XCHL48), under the aegis of their 'Nations and Regions' programme, and part of the 'Constitutional Change and Identity' project convened by Professor David McCrone of Edinburgh University. I am very grateful to Dr Francine Lorimer for her comments, also to Dr Frances Rapport and the audience at the New Qualitative Methodology seminar, University of Wales, Swansea.

Notes

1 With the permission of the hospital authorities (the Chief Executive and the Dean, to whom I wrote), the portering charge-hands and union (to whom the hospital authorities then spoke), I undertook, in a voluntary capacity, the day-to-day shiftwork of a porter over a period of nine months. I hoped as far as possible to insinuate myself into a porter's life-world at Constance Hospital (and, to a lesser extent, outside the hospital too) by doing as and what other porters did.
2 'Social anthropology' was the name of the discipline that developed in Britain during the twentieth century and 'cultural anthropology' that in North America. Due to the growth of professional centres of anthropology (continental Europe, Australasia, Israel, India) and the increasing overlap in their enterprises – encompassing both an appreciation of social structure and the institutional, and the provenance of the symbological – the convention has grown to refer, as I do here, to 'sociocultural anthropology'.
3 For a discussion of these terms, as against the 'positivistic' or 'naturalistic', see Giddens (1974) and Wolff (1978).
4 For elaboration on the range of methods anthropologists employ, see Ellen (1984), or Bernard (1998). For discussion of participant observation in particular, its history, ethics, biography and recent developments, see Spindler (1970), Okely and Callaway (1992), Rapport (1993: 69–77), Michrina and Richards (1996), Aull Davies (1998), and Amit (1999).
5 My fieldwork practice was not to tape-record informants but yet to aim for a detailed accounting of interactions I witnessed. As soon as possible after an interaction's end I would therefore discreetly transcribe key words onto paper, for a full writing-up in my journal later.

References

Allport, G. (1942) *The Use of Personal Documents in Psychological Science*, New York: Social Science Research Council.

Amit, V., ed., (1999) *Constructing the Field*, London: Routledge.

Aull Davies, C. (1998) *Reflexive Ethnography*, London: Routledge.

Bernard, H., ed., (1998) *Handbook of Methods in Cultural Anthropology*, Walnut Creek, CA: Altamira.

Cohen, A. P. (1994) *Self Consciousness*, London: Routledge.

Dumont, J-P. (1978) *The Headman and I*, Austin: University of Texas Press.

Ellen, R., ed., (1984) *Ethnographic Research*, London: Academic Press.

Forster, E. M. (1984) *Aspects of the Novel*, Harmondsworth: Penguin.

Geertz, C. (1983) *Local Knowledge*, New York: Basic Publishing.

Giddens, A., ed., (1974) *Positivism and Sociology*, London: Heinemann.

Goodman, N. (1978) *Ways of Worldmaking*, Hassocks, E.Sussex: Harvester.

Ingold, T., ed., (1997) *Key Debates in Anthropology*, London: Routledge.

Lambert, H. and McKevitt, C. (2002) 'Anthropology in health research: From qualitative methods to multidisciplinarity', *British Medical Journal,* 325: 210–12.

Leach, E. R. (1982) *Social Anthropology*, London: Fontana.

Leach, E. R. (1984) 'Glimpses of the unmentionable in the history of British social anthropology', *Annual Review of Anthropology,* 13: 1–23.

Leach, E. R. (1989) 'Writing anthropology: A review of Geertz's *Works and Lives*', *American Ethnologist,* 16(1): 137–41.

Louch, A. (1966) *Explanation and Human Action*, Oxford: Blackwell.

Michrina, B. and Richards, C. (1996) *Person to Person*, Albany: State University of New York Press.

Needham, R. (1978) *Primordial Characters*, Charlottesville: University of Virginia Press.

Nietzsche, F. (1911) 'On truth and falsity in their ultramoral sense (1873)', in *Early Greek Philosophy, and Other Essays*. London: Foulis.

Okely, J. and Callaway, H., eds, (1992), *Anthropology and Autobiography*, London: Routledge.

Prigogine, I. (1989) 'The philosophy of instability', *Futures,* August: 396–400.

Rapport, N. J. (1993) *Diverse World-Views in an English Village*, Edinburgh: Edinburgh University Press.

Rapport, N. J. (1994) *The Prose and the Passion: Anthropology, Literature and the Writing of E. M. Forster*, Manchester: Manchester University Press.

Rapport, N. J. (1997a) 'Opposing the motion that "Cultural Studies will be the Death of Anthropology"', *Group for Debates in Anthropological Theory*, Department of Social Anthropology, University of Manchester.

Rapport, N. J. (1997b) *Transcendent Individual: Towards a Liberal and Literary Anthropology*, London: Routledge.

Rapport, N. J. (2002) '"The truth is alive": Kierkegaard's anthropology of subjectivism, dualism and somatic knowledge', *Anthropological Theory,* 2(2): 165–83.

Spindler, G., ed., (1970) *Being an Anthropologist*, New York: Holt, Rinehart and Winston.

Turner, V. (1982) *The Ritual Process*, Ithaca: Cornell University Press.

Wagner, R. (1977) 'Culture as creativity', in Dolgin, J., Kemnitzer, D. and Schneider, D., eds, *Symbolic Anthropology*, New York: Columbia University Press.

Wolff, K. (1978) 'Phenomenology and Sociology', in Bottomore, T. and Nisbet R., eds, *A History of Sociological Analysis*, New York: Basic Publishing.

Chapter 6

Imagework method and potential applications in health, social sciences and social care research

Journeying with a question

Iain Edgar

My dearest friend, how much longer must I watch you shrinking, diminishing before my eyes. How long will it be before you can accept that you are well again, that the operation was a success and that which you most fear has gone, has been excised. Your body is whole again, you are well – but you are not healed. You stay in this house, day after day, living with the physical scars which should be a symbol of new life, but for you they are the mark of death. You must come out of the dark and the cold, you must feel again the warmth and joy of living, you must come with me, for I am going to take you on a journey to a place of healing. It will be easy, you have only to take a few steps, out of this place, and be free.

You see, it wasn't too hard. It is beautiful, the sun is gathering strength and soon it will be hot, with blue skies – a perfect day. Now that you are outside we can begin our journey. It will be no ordinary journey, you must think of it as a 'magic carpet ride'.

The above is an extract from a participant's write-up of an imagework journey conducted with a group of social anthropology students. I introduced the exercise in a handout as follows:

Imagework has variously been called 'active imagination', 'visualisation' and 'guided fantasy'. Imagework is also a powerful therapeutic method, as described by Glouberman (1989) and Achterberg (1985). Imagework has developed from the active imagination technique of Jung and the theory and practice of psychosynthesis developed by Assagioli (1965). Jung's (1959: 42) concept of the 'collective unconscious' underpins imagework. The concept of the 'collective unconscious' represented Jung's perception that the human psyche contained impersonal and archaic contents that manifested themselves in the myths, dreams and images of humans. Jung's idea that all humans contained a common and universal storehouse of psychic contents, which he called 'archetypes', is the core model of the unconscious that enables imagework practitioners (see Glouberman 1989: 25) to consider the spontaneous image as being potentially a creative and emergent aspect of the self. The imagework method is an active process in which the person 'actively imagining' lets go of the mind's normal train of thoughts and images and goes with a sequence of imagery that arises spontaneously from the unconscious. It is the quality of spontaneity and unexpectedness that are the hallmarks of this process. Imagework has creative potential because as Clandinin writes:

> In this view, images are seen as the mediator between the unconscious and conscious levels of being. What is known at the unconscious level finds expression in a person's thought and actions through a person's images. Images are thus seen as the source of inspiration, ideas, insight and meaning.
>
> (Clandinin 1986: 17)

Of course, all the time we are 'doing' imagework: 'anticipating, rehearsing; "going over things", remembering, daydreaming ... dreaming ... in short we are visualisers as well as thinkers and feelers ...' (Edgar 1999: 199). Imagework can elicit/facilitate more implicit, less conscious, ideas that we have, drawing on our intuitive and affective (emotional) aspects, as well as our cognitive/rational processes.

> (Workshop handout)

The workshop then continued as follows:

TUTOR: We will first do a relaxation exercise: for its own sake but also to become 'more in touch' with our right-brain hemisphere, which deals with our creativity, intuitions and emotions ...

OK then: first relax ... breath deeply ... or imagine a safe place ... or let your awareness travel through your body ...

Then when you are ready ... imagine meeting your friend, say at a railway station or somewhere ... you are going to take them to a 'therapeutic' or healing place ... now in your own time: make that journey ... share what is happening with them ... now you are reaching the place ... what does it look like? Knock on the door! You are greeted ... then you go in ... what's it like? ... have a good look round ... introduce your friend ... then just spend some time there ... explore ... Now you are going to leave ... with or without your friend

... say your goodbyes and return to whence you came! Come back into the room ...

Now briefly, make a little coloured picture of your imaginative experience ... enjoy doing it ... share the whole experience with a friend ... or two ... use your picture as a means of sharing ...

Masks could be made from these journeys; dances and little dramas enacted; the possibilities are almost endless.

Further questions can be asked of these 'inner journeys', depending on whether the objectives are personal growth related, education orientated (see Edgar forthcoming) or qualitative research in design. The use of imagework for qualitative health and social care research is the focus of this paper.

My interest in developing an imagework exercise that consists of taking participants and their 'needy friend' to a healing community or 'place' in their imagination grew from several roots. These included recently visiting a medical sociologist friend and colleague, who had had a psychotic breakdown, in a local inpatient psychiatric facility and witnessing their perception of this facility as being profoundly anti-therapeutic. Such a perception is confirmed by the outcome of the Sainsbury Centre (1998) study of such facilities.

Later I participated in developing a multidisciplinary research proposal to consider service users' perceptions of their desired change. Working towards such ends necessitated eliciting service users' ideal picture of a therapeutic environment. Since then I have developed this imagework exercise as a way of developing and accessing participants' intuitive views of their ideal therapeutic environment (although the 'journey' format is one in which the participant is apparently taking a 'needy friend' to a therapeutic place, of course really it is their own vision of such a place). I first worked with a group of mature German cultural studies students for a day and was very surprised by what I found. Most of the students developed a very politically Green perspective, with their healing places located away from the city and in the country, often with water nearby, such as a lake. Access to friends was central, as was developing a self-structuring programme for the day; psychiatrists and pills were nowhere in sight! Of course, a critical perspective on the results of this day workshop would say that these were probably radical German students and what did you expect! Since then, however, I have done this exercise with several non-National Health Service patient groups and have continued to be surprised by the themes that arise in these journeys. Nature imagery is paramount generally; beauty has a definite place in peoples' constructions and oftentimes I have wondered whether I am triggering or facilitating some kind of paradisical mini-archetype latent in human consciousness, rather like Newberg and d'Aquili (1994) suggest in relation to their research on the universality of near-death experiences. Certainly participants usually report very calming experiences and often meetings with significant others, such as a dearly loved and departed grandparent. Indeed, one of the slight issues with using imagework is that participants can use the opportunity to 'do' unfinished business rather than focusing on the instructions given. The following is such a case.

> Then suddenly we were in this huge soap-bubble and we were suspended above the countryside, we were gliding through the air. Inside of the soap-bubble were lots of fluffy feathers. It was calm up there, it felt like being sheltered, a place to rest, to take breath, there was clearness, facility, lots of wideness ... just being away from real world. I held the girl in my arms and we stayed there for the rest of the 'journey' gliding through the air. Actually it was me who enjoyed this quiet, peacefully place the most ... just being there was the healing aspect.

The participant's comments on the exercise were as follows:[1]

> That day we made this 'journey' I didn't feel well. I had a lot of things on my mind, I was stressed out ... I guess that's why I immediately found myself in this wonderful soap-bubble without any friend who needed help ... I guess I myself needed urgently such a place and that's why I stayed there for the rest of the exercise! That morning the healing place of the 'journey' was a real healing place for me.

For the participant this was clearly a 'healing' experience and she did have a child companion; she says, however, that she 'immediately found herself in this wonderful soap-bubble without any friend who needs help'. I often find that participants don't follow the instructions exactly as they may have more pressing needs for personal peace, etc. This is not a problem, though, as many participants will 'do the journey' exactly as asked and from slightly different journeys experienced, such as the above, perhaps new valuable insights may later emerge when analysing the data generated. The priority is that participants meet their own needs and feel safe and experience the exercise as personally valuable. From such experiences personal meaning and a vision of self can emerge.

Such results show that many people have an innate, intuitive vision of what for them is a healing place and these visions seem rarely to be available as a reality in the statutory sector. Indeed, some of the recent literature on inpatient psychiatric care seems to focus less on developing a therapeutic environment and more on avoiding suicide (Bongar et al. 1998), violence (Royal College of Psychiatrists 1998) or sexual harassment (National Health Service Executive 1997). Whilst Utopian or visionary perspectives may suffer from a certain lack of political and financial realism, they do stimulate the debate and provide benchmarks as to what people and service users actually believe and hope for. As such, they are ironically foundational to any study of local stakeholders' perceptions of appropriate change, and without such elicited views how will service users relate to NHS and/or psychiatric service agendas for change?

Imagework and the qualitative research domain

So far social science research has barely begun to utilise such powerful strategies as imagework which were developed originally for personal and group change but which are potentially applicable to qualitative research. This chapter will locate these methods within the qualitative research domain and propose a novel view of their value. Even the second edition of the *Handbook of Qualitative Research* (Denzin and Lincoln 2000) makes almost no mention of these methods. The chapter in the original 1994 edition on 'personal experience methods' refers only to journals, diaries, annals, storytelling and so forth (Clandinin and Connelly 1994). Nor do these methods seem to appear in even advanced focus group methods (Fern 2001). Only Stuhlmiller and Thorsen (1997: 140–9), separately, report on their use through a related method that they call 'narrative picturing'. Participatory research activities use many experiential exercises, but as far as I know have not integrated imagework as a practice into their methodologies (Pretty *et al.* 1995). Recently some uses of imagework and dreaming have emerged in the transpersonal research methods field of psychology (Braud and Anderson 1998). Transpersonal psychology, as Anderson writes:

> seeks to delve deeply into the most profound and inexplicable aspects of human experiences, including mystical and unitive experiences, experiences of transformation, extraordinary insight, meditative awareness, altered states of consciousness, and self-actualisation.
>
> (Anderson 1998: 69)

Anderson calls this approach 'intuitive enquiry' and advocates the acknowledged use of:

> various altered states of consciousness, active dreaming and dream incubation, mystical vision and audition, intentional imaging, kinaesthetic and somatic awareness, and states of consciousness more typically associated with the artistic process than with science, in all phases of the enquiry.
>
> (Anderson 1998: 76)

Whilst imagework may be seen as a potential research method in transpersonal psychology, my exploration of imagework as a research methodology has shown that its value is potentially located across the broad qualitative research field, particularly qualitative health and social care research. The hypothesis underpinning my imagework approach is that experiential research methods, such as imagework, can elicit and evoke implicit knowledge and self-identities of respondents in a way that other methods cannot.

Imaginary fields

There are several different kinds or fields of imagework. Imagework can be as simple as asking respondents, individually or in a group, to imagine an image in response to a question, such as 'How do you picture a certain situation?' I shall call this first field *'introductory imagework'*. A second field of imagework involves guiding respondents into their memory of earlier events, such as their childhood socialisation. I call this second field *'memory imagework'*. A third field of imagework, such as the 'healing places' exercise, involves the use of the Jungian active imagination technique, which facilitates a spontaneous journey into the imagination. I define this field as *'spontaneous imagework'*.

Imagework and dreamwork are very closely related and in certain ways overlap, in that both refer to the mind's spontaneous production of imagery that people may consider is 'good to think with'. This fourth field of imagework I shall refer to as *'dream imagework'*. The historical, cross-cultural and contemporary use of dreams for diagnosis and healing constitutes a vast arena going back to at least Assyrian and ancient Egyptian dreamwork practices, and particularly the ancient Greek temple healing dream incubation methods described by Artimedorus (Mackenzie 1965). However, dreamwork per se is not the focus of this paper but will be covered substantially as part of an overall imagework methodology in my forthcoming book (Edgar forthcoming).

The analytic processing of imagework into data can have up to four stages: first, the descriptive stage wherein respondents 'tell their story'; second, analysis by participants of the personal meaning of their experience of symbols used; third, analysis of the models used to inform their imagery; and fourth, the comparative stage when respondents compare their imagework with that of others in the group. Each of these stages needs facilitation and can be promoted through the amplification of the imagework into art and drama.

In using an experiential method such as imagework, it is also important to realise that while in itself imagework is a largely non-verbal activity, it produces a verbal communication that incorporates the respondents' interpretations. Therefore, a respondent explaining the results of their imagework will typically relate a verbal account of their experience to the group, including the researcher. The results of imagework become a verbal communication capable of transcription and so becoming a 'field text' (Clandinin and Connelly 1994) for the researcher.

Apart from the 'bowl of soup' exercise outlined later, I shall not focus on the first field of introductory imagework. I refer the interested reader to Edgar (1999).

Memory imagework

Memory imagework exercises can be focused on health themes. An exercise I often do is to ask respondents to recollect or remember their life with respect to experiences of health and illness as a way of finding out differential models of health and wellbeing held by certain groups. As part of the exercise, respondents also have to fill in a set of accompanying questions that relate to their memory exercise.

As an example, I will consider one case where the respondent drew a picture of a tree with energy centres along it, culminating in a bird sitting at the top of the tree. At first sight the picture hardly seems to resemble anything much to do with health, until the respondent's explanation of their symbolic construction is read. I will report in full the answers to the following questions:

Q: How did you visualise your life?
A: As a tree; with many branches and experiences, still growing and learning. The tree's roots also represent strong family roots and a stable basis upon which to grow and rely. The tree, growing towards the sky is also symbolic of my ambitions and dreams for the future.

Q: What critical incidents did you remember?
A: Death.

Q: What 'health' issues came up?
A: Stress, pain, headaches initially, but flowing into peace, contentment and happiness.

Q: How did you portray health-related issues? What symbols did you use to show 'healthy' and 'unhealthy' times?
A: Weather-related symbols were used because I feel they are very accurate in portraying emotions felt when going through good times (sunshine) and bad times (lightning). The sleeping bird represents the future goal of ultimate contentment in life.

Q: How was/is our experience of 'health' affected by the society we live in?
A: Remembering mostly the bad times rather than the good; coming from a Western society, our experience of health is more focused towards the physical being: fitness, appearance; traditionally putting much less emphasis on the health of the spirit.

Q: As an observer looking at your picture what do you see?
A: The use of symbols from Western culture – very general symbols encompassing good and bad times with death (cross) being the only independent symbol and therefore obviously the most important issue.

Q: What ideas about health can be seen in the picture?
A: The idea that the good and the bad times are linked, one following on from another. That both are needed in order to grow and reach contentment.

We can deduce from an examination of the picture and transcripts, perhaps, the following health themes and perspectives emerging from the exercise and resulting symbolism. This picture, in common with many of the others from the exercise, shows a marked capacity for symbolism to express individual perceptions of health 'careers'. The tree symbol itself is a powerful and cross-cultural metaphor through which to express the nature of a human being. The world tree is a well-known symbol. Other symbols evoked through the exercise are the sleeping bird, sunshine and lightning. It is very common for participants to describe healthy times through positive meteorological symbols, and inversely, to use symbolic images such as rain and cloud to portray negative times. Likewise, metaphors of 'ascent' and 'descent' are often used, as when the participant says, referring to the tree, 'growing towards the sky is also a symbolic image to express hope, ambitions and dreams for the future'. A similar symbol used in the same exercise by another participant was a series of hills, with ascents for 'healthy times' and descents expressing 'unhealthy times', and yet another participant drew on the symbolism of a rollercoaster. The use of such symbolisation allows participants to empathise with one another without having to disclose possibly confidential health data.

However, what I consider valuable about the depth of the data revealed through these examples are the many levels of understanding of health that emerge. Unlike in some of Seedhouse's (1986) four theories of health, we can 'see' an individual's metaphorical account of their remembered and also deeply anticipated future hopes. Moreover, these thoughts, feelings and aspirations are couched in a visually expressed narrative that encompasses 'stress, pain, headaches initially but flowing into peace, contentment and happiness' (Seedhouse 1986: 51–4). Health becomes much more than pain, illness and disease episodes and includes social relationships and the thread of meaning running through the participant's life and even projected into their future. This account is more akin to a humanistic and holistic view of health than to other Western theories of health. All the participants' pictures are unique, but they often utilise common symbolism (metaphors of ascent and descent for good and bad times, for example). The pictures are open to varying levels of analysis and meta-analysis, as previously described. The data obtained is imaginatively evoked as much as thought and so the data obtained is more holistic in the sense that it can and often does draw on the affective and intuitive aspects of the self as well as the rational.

Spontaneous imagework

Spontaneous imagework, which was the third of my four fields, is the main focus of this chapter. As we have seen in the first 'healing places' exercise, spontaneous imagework consists of leading a group of respondents on an imaginary journey. Examples of these journeys are written up in Ernst and Goodison (1981), Glouberman (1989) and Markham (1989). A typical exercise of this type is for the facilitator, after an introductory relaxation exercise, to lead the participants on a journey. A classical form of this is to start the journey in a meadow and to lead participants over an obstacle and up a hill to a house where they meet a wise person whom they can talk to about any question that they have. An exercise like this (Ernst and Goodison, 1981: 161), in my experience, can trigger disclosure of and work on important personal, health and social issues. For qualitative research purposes, this kind of exercise can be refocused to gain data concerning the subject of an enquiry. So, for example, if the researcher wished to gain data about respondents' views on any aspect of family life or social life, they would be asked to 'carry' this question in their mind and ask their 'wise old person' about this subject.

One recent imagework exercise I have adapted for use from Glouberman's 'sensing life choices, making life decisions' (1989: 168–86) I call 'crossroads'. In this exercise I suggest that participants first develop a question about their life that currently is of interest to them; the question can be either a small or a large one. Then they imagine the choices they have with respect to this question and I ask them, following a suitable relaxation exercise, to visualise the different ways or paths that the different choices would offer. They then 'walk' down those different ways and encounter often surprising material that, subsequently in discussion, they can relate to their intuitive expectation of life outcomes following particular decisions. Sometimes, as a variant on this exercise, participants can towards the end imagine themselves going up in a helicopter or a balloon above the different 'paths' and see for themselves how the ways come together later or veer away from each other. Perhaps they all lead to the same place anyway!

How can this exercise be used in a research context? Well, any research question that involves the issue of health and personal and contextual decision-making, or risk assessment, is an obvious topic. People's perception of impending life changes and their expected and unexpected coping capacities and resources manifest themselves well through such an exercise and probably in differing ways from a purely conceptual discussion. Participants can, for instance, visualise different courses of action, and their imagined outcomes (costs and benefits), in relation to healthy and unhealthy lifestyles, relationship and career issues. Issues such as perceptions of pregnancy, marriage, divorce, bereavement and even death (end of life choices) could be conjured up and worked with. Imagework exercises offer the opportunity to pull together the social context with biomedicine. As well as a focus on health sector consumers, a 'crossroads' imagework exercise can offer professional health workers opportunities to assess and value differing priorities in health investment and treatment options.

It is worth considering that we all anticipate and rehearse our possible futures during a large part of our daytime life, and possibly in our dreamtime too. We anticipate the day or evening or weekend ahead; where we might go on holiday if time and money permitted; whom we might try and date or make friends with. In all these activities and countless others we are normally engaged in, we – excepting those few who are not visual thinkers at all – imaginatively predict the possible outcomes, so that in an informal way, we do the 'crossroads' exercise many times each day, but usually we do it in a haphazard and somewhat undisciplined form and of course normally we do our imaginative rehearsal work on our own or 'chewing it' over with a friend.

Ethical and practical issues

Clearly the use of the different fields of the imagework method require familiarity with their use and skill in their application, though arguably a researcher could observe an imagework practitioner using such a method, rather than using it her/himself. Care over use is important as such a method can reveal latent feelings and unrealised intuitions that have often previously only been partially conscious or possibly even repressed. However, specific training programmes in these hitherto 'therapeutic' methods do now exist.[2] Moreover, introductory imagework is not difficult to use. A couple of training sessions with colleagues and a facilitator should suffice. I usually start a workshop session with the following exercise:

Introductory exercise: bowl of soup or 'in the soup'!

The aim of the exercise is to show that the 'unconscious' mind is always accessible – like a well of images awaiting our attention. The primary intention of this exercise is as a warm-up to longer imagework exercises. This exercise can be used to give a symbolic view on a person's current self-state, though I tend not to focus on this aspect.

1   Ask students to imagine themselves drinking in silence a bowl of soup; alternatively this 'imaginary' bowl could be passed round a group (I prefer this option).
2   Give people a couple of minutes to imagine the bowl of soup; make sure people have been asked not to giggle beforehand.

3   Then ask two or three people to share: (a) what was the soup? (b) what was the bowl?

Typically, there is quite a variety of responses: one person 'flew' through the bottom of the bowl into a mountain range (an experienced traveller); others remembered a 'favourite soup' which had a particular meaning for them. One respondent spoke of a 'champagne and pea' soup! Half-empty bowls can illustrate feelings of not being fed enough (I remember a mother who said she always focused on feeding others, hence her bowl was half empty). Often there is a split between those who imagine their bowls with home-made (often mother's or grandmother's) soup, which has overtones of family nurturing etc., and those who have tinned soup. This contrast is 'good to work with'. Or the bowl itself can be of interest and is often 'special' to the person in some way: meanings and associations can be developed here. For example a manager's bowl of soup was a very large bowl with a ladle and many smaller bowls! Sometimes a part of a person's life journey can be symbolised, as when an anthropologist combined in her soup images the tastes and textures of her European homeland with the smells of her African fieldwork setting.

The 'bowl of soup' exercise shows how quickly the unconscious throws up an image or a set of images. Moreover, these images can be read – albeit not always easily – as intuitively relevant picturings of some aspect of the person's life at that time, the 'exhausted' mother, e.g. the deserted mother? Using such an introductory imagework exercise at the beginning of a workshop session reassures participants and allows them to identify with the imagework process. Such practice is part of a sensitive and ethical imagework practice.

The ethics of imagework

The ethics of using imagework approaches are important. An imagework methodology should only be practised within accepted social science ethical guidelines. Christians (2001: 138–40) summarises the main codes of ethics for professional and academic qualitative research communities as consisting of four main guidelines: informed consent, opposition to deception, privacy and confidentiality, and accuracy. Any research activity using imagework and its associated techniques should meet normative requirements in these areas. Informed consent requirements can be met through the careful explanation of the processes to be involved, though it is important to note what Parse (1995: 82) has called 'lingering true presence' (see overleaf). Deception is obviously important to avoid, whereas normal expectations of privacy and confidentiality can be maintained and are especially important in research activity that aims to elicit 'deep' data from respondents. Accurancy is likewise equally important.

Clearly some researchers will feel that the imagework method is unacceptably intrusive and raises power issues that are very problematic. However, whilst I would propose that an experiential method such as imagework has as its intention the gathering of in-depth data, I would argue that any data collection method involves intrusion and can provoke problems of self-disclosure. Even a simple interview can suddenly trigger a sensitive area for the respondent and leave the researcher with ethical considerations in terms of how to handle the resulting situation supportively. Johnson and Griffith (1998: 212) suggest that all interviewing technologies are primarily concerned with enabling respondents to 'open up', particularly with respect to complex concerns. Some ethnographic methods, such as photo-elicitation in particular, seek in a similar way to open up the respondent to dimly perceived or remembered emotional depths (Collier 1967: 67). The methods I have outlined will sometimes be a catalyst for significant disclosure, yet the negative aspects of disclosure can be greatly prevented by making participation voluntary, by the sensitive explanation of the task and technique to participants beforehand, and by similar aftercare. Moreover, participants can be asked again, following an imagework exercise, if they wish their contribution to be used as part of the research findings.

It is important to be aware that the creative, emotional and cognitive influence of an image may not be completed within the timespan of the session. Parse, as part of her 'human becoming theory,' has called this after-effect 'lingering true presence' (1995: 82). The evocative power of a symbol may engage the mind in an ongoing process of self-enquiry; therefore it may be prudent for the researcher, as well as ensuring that their respondents finish the task at ease with any imaginative results, to make follow-up individual or group interviews available.

Some topics may be inappropriate for imagework, certainly in groups, and there is an appropriate literature on researching sensitive issues that is relevant to the use of imagework methods (Renzetti and Lee 1993). However, one advantage of using imagework, and often following up with artwork, is that it enables respondents to discuss potentially sensitive material in a coded way that allows them to retain their privacy. People can, for instance, verbally or in their accompanying artwork, refer to 'bad times' by using stereotypical images of unhappiness such as 'bad weather' and, as a result, retain their privacy and their understanding of their meaning.

Guidelines for safe practice

- Explain everything beforehand: go through each part of the exercise, so there are no surprises along the way.
- Give clear permission to people that they don't have to do the session if they don't want to.

- After introducing the exercise and before doing it, ask 'Any questions?'.
- Develop trust from the beginning, using open body gestures and clear, quiet voice tone. Reassure participants continually that 'they' are in control throughout the exercise and included during the sharing – it is their journey.
- Plan the timing of the session and allow enough time for each part of it – don't try and do too much. Go through each part of the session in your mind beforehand. Prepare yourself.
- Pace the visualisation process by doing the visualisation yourself at the same time as the people you are facilitating. Make sure you leave plenty of time during the visualisation for people's imaginations to work.
- Practise with friends/colleagues beforehand, if you wish.
- If you feel really unsure about doing this exercise, as opposed to your 'normal' level of apprehension before doing a new type of exercise, then either don't do it or choose a safer format.
- Talk through with respondents 'self-care' issues first. Emphasise that they are in control of all parts of the process. They can guarantee their confidentiality by what they choose to share with others. Point out that symbols have many meanings and associations, and their multivocality is a real asset for both eliciting ideas and retaining confidentiality.
- If respondents are unhappy, ill, worried or preoccupied, advise them not to do the exercise, or particularly to look after themselves.
- Advise people that if they become distracted in an exercise then they can gently bring their wandering attention back to the subject.
- If someone encounters a 'difficult' memory or image, advise them that they have a choice either to go on with the exercise or to stop and imagine something more pleasant. However, remind them that their images and accompanying feelings and thoughts are theirs. Also, be clear that difficult feelings can also be triggered by 'outer' events, for instance the look or smell of a flower. This subject of difficult memory/image recall can be gone into in more depth and discussion facilitated as to the possible long-term value of dealing with difficult memories that can suddenly intrude into consciousness; is the 'unconscious' good at timing in all cases?
- Don't allow any interruptions during the session: put a very clear message on the door and even an object like a chair to block late entrants!
- Facilitate everyone sharing their feelings and experiences that have been evoked by the exercise, at least in pairs, so that each person has had the opportunity to tell 'their' story.
- Be available after the session, or ensure a colleague is around, to provide support if needed – though in my experience this is rare. Watch carefully to see if anyone is looking upset at the end.

Conclusion

Here is the end of the participant's journey started at the beginning of this chapter:

> Now I can look back on that time and I can see how it was – the advent of your healing. I can see now that it was necessary for you to take that first step, a step that signalled your intention to return to life. It was necessary for you to go somewhere safe and familiar – and what better place could there be than a summer garden. It was necessary for the mind to be filled with beautiful, living, fragrant images, for your lungs to be filled with pure, clean air, for your soul to be filled with hope.

So the thesis of this chapter is that a 'new' research methodology such as imagework offers the opportunity for researchers to further study the personal and social world of the respondent and so obtain a blend of cognitive, affective and intuitive material known, dimly known, implicit, suppressed and even repressed by the conscious mind. Overall, the chapter has shown the way that imagework, one of several potential experiential research methods, offers researchers the means to access the latent knowledge and unexpressed feelings of respondents.

This chapter has partly provided a detailed guide for the beginning practitioner of the imagework method; also, it has suggested a way forward for imagework practice as a part of the research process in the health and social care arenas, and it has outlined a basic typological framework for imagework practitioners/researchers. Experiential research methods such as imagework can be utilised in part or on their own in research practice in such diverse fields as health and social care, social sciences, education, development and even business and marketing. The imagework method is particularly effective in accessing participants' implicit awareness of such areas as individual and collective vision development; personal and cultural identity formation and change; interpersonal dynamics, attitudes and ideologies; and organisational culture. While the application of the imagework method may be considered innovative, the principles, ethics and practices governing the organisation and analysis of data derived from this method remain firmly within the established qualitative domain. The way is open for further studies using these methods, perhaps in controlled and cross-cultural studies that would compare the value of such experiential methods against the use of more traditional research methods.

Overall in this chapter I argue, with suggestive examples from my own imagework groups, that imagination-based research methods constitute a coherent research practice. Moreover, imagework as a particular research practice can be related to and integrated with other innovative research methods, such as transpersonal (Braud and Anderson 1998), participatory (Pretty *et al.* 1995) and other arts-based research methods (Norris and Buck 2002).

Notes

1 I have run imagework groups with a wide range of participants: researchers, educators, students and others; consent to use examples of participants' 'journeys' has been explicitly obtained.
2 I occasionally run training courses; I am aware of an imagework training agency based in California that offers distance and personal training in the use of 'interactive guided imagery'(http://www.interactiveimagery.com). I have no direct experience of it.

References

Achterberg, J. (1985) *Imagery in Healing*, Boston: Shambhala.

Anderson, R. (1998) 'Intuitive inquiry', in Baud, W. and Anderson R., eds, *Transpersonal Research Methods for the Social Sciences*, London: Sage Publications.

Assagioli, R. (1965) *Psychosynthesis*, London: Mandala and Psychosynthesis Research Foundation.

Bongar, B., Berman, A., Maris, R., Silverman, M., Harris, E. and Packman, W. (1998) *Risk Management with Suicidal Patients*, New York: Guildford.

Braud, W. and Anderson, R. (1998) *Transpersonal Research Methods for the Social Sciences*, London: Sage Publications.

Christians, C. (2001) 'Ethics and politics in qualitative research', in Denzin, G. and Lincoln, Y., eds, *Handbook of Qualitative Research*, London: Sage Publications.

Clandinin, D. (1986). *Classroom Practice: Teacher Images in Action*, London: Falmer Press.

Clandinin, D. and Connelly, F. (1994) 'Personal experience methods', in Denzin, N. and Lincoln, Y., eds, *Handbook of Qualitative Research*, London: Sage Publications.

Collier, J. (1967) *Visual Anthropology: Photography as a Research Method*, New York: Holt, Rinehart and Winston.

Denzin, N. and Lincoln, Y. (1994) *Handbook of Qualitative Research*, London: Sage Publications.

Denzin, N. and Lincoln, Y. (2000) *Handbook of Qualitative Research*, 2nd edn, London: Sage Publications.

Edgar, I. (1999) 'The imagework method in social science and health research', *Qualitative Health Research*, 9 (2): 198–211.

Edgar, I. (forthcoming) *Guide to Imagework: Imagination-Based Research Methods*, London: Routledge.

Ernst, S. and Goodison, L. (1981) *In Our Own Hands: A Book of Self-Help Therapy*, London: The Women's Press.

Fern, E. (2001) *Advanced Focus Group Research*, Newbury Park, CA: Sage Publications.

Glouberman, D. (1989) *Life Choices and Life Changes Through Imagework*, London: Unwin.

Johnson, J. and Griffith, D. (1998) 'Visual data: Collection, analysis and representation', in de Munck, V. and Sobo E., eds, *Using Methods in the Field: A Practical Introduction and Casebook*, Walnut Creek, CA: Altamira Press.

Jung, C. (1959) 'Archetypes of the collective unconscious,' in *The Collected Works of C. G. Jung* 9, 1, London: Routledge and Kegan Paul.

Mackenzie, N. (1965) *Dreams and Dreaming*, London: Aldus Books.

Markham, U. (1989) *The Elements of Visualisation*, Shaftesbury, Dorset: Element Books.

National Health Service Executive (1997) *Summary of Health Authorities' Target Dates to Secure Acceptable Standards of Segregated Hospital Accommodation*, London: National Health Service Executive.

Newberg, A. and d'Aquili, E. (1994) 'The NDE as archetype: A model for "prepared" neurocognitive processes', *Anthropology of Consciousness*, 5, 4: 1–15.

Norris, J. and Buck, G. (2002) 'Editorial' in Theme Issue: Exemplars of arts-based research methodologies, *Alberta Journal of Educational Research*, XLV111, (3) Fall: 203–5.

Parse, R. (1995) 'The human becoming practice methodology', in Parse, R., ed., *Illuminations: The Human Becoming Theory in Practice and Research*, New York: National League for Nursing Press.

Pretty, J., Gujit, I., Thompson, J. and Scoones, I. (1995) *A Trainer's Guide for Participatory Learning and Action*, London: International Institute for Environment and Development.

Renzetti, C. and Lee, R. (1993) *Researching Sensitive Topics*, Newbury Park, CA: Sage Publications.

Royal College of Psychiatrists (1998) *The Management of Violence in Clinical Settings: An Evidence-Based Guideline*, London: Royal College of Psychiatrists Research Support Unit.

Sainsbury Centre for Mental Health (1998) *Acute Problems – A Survey of the Quality of Care in Acute Psychiatric Wards*, London: Sainsbury Centre for Mental Health.

Seedhouse, D. (1986) *Health: The Foundations for Achievement*, Chichester, W. Sussex: John Wiley.

Stuhlmiller, C. and Thorsen, R. (1997) 'Narrative picturing: A new strategy for qualitative data collection', *Qualitative Health Research*, 7, 1: 140–9.

Chapter 7

Postmodern literary poetics of experience

A new form of aesthetic enquiry

Francis C. Biley

Anybody who stumbles into the world of research, and perhaps in particular healthcare research, could be forgiven for thinking that there were only a certain number of different approaches that could be taken, and that there is a fairly well defined battery of traditional methods that can be employed to examine areas of concern. An examination of any of the standard research textbooks will reveal rigorous and clear explorations and explanations of existing methods, from the perceived objective reality of statistically based randomised controlled trials and surveys to qualitative designs that may encompass, but are not limited to, ethnography, phenomenology, action research, historiography, grounded theory and so on. In recent years the significance of the Kantian notion of the importance of a perceived and dynamic (rather than an actual and static) reality appears to be in the ascendancy, and the aforementioned research methods are receiving increasing scrutiny and use in order to explore meaning. However, if the idea of individually perceived dynamic realities, with multiple interpretations of any kind of material that we are encountering, is pursued to its logical conclusion, then there is a need to question the very nature of any form of research, even that known as 'qualitative'. The legitimacy of objective science and its occupation with explaining observed phenomena and cause and effect relationships can be questioned, but so can the science that proclaims to explore meaning and dynamic realities because, paradoxically, they are limited by the social context of their existence and the absolute and objective qualities of the language with which we choose to communicate a/the dynamic reality. In other words, taking the concept or perspective of the 'incredulity of metanarratives' (Lyotard 1984: 24), we simply cannot describe a dynamic reality using language systems that are static and claim, by their very existence, to be objective.

We need to break down existing language and communication systems, such as the printed and spoken word, representative paintings and three-dimensional sculpture and music, pushing beyond the fabricated quantitative–qualitative continuum into the realm of the aesthetic, in order to discover or reveal new realities.

In this chapter I aim to explore one way of achieving this, describing the development of one method of inquiry that may be called aesthetic rather than scientific, by calling on the work not of those philosophers and theorists who would normally inform research practice, but a group of radically creative individuals who became known as the 'Beat Generation', and in particular, William S. Burroughs.

The Beat Generation

Although a very speculative claim, it would seem to make sense that the creative arts and literature movement that began in New York during the 1940s and lasted through the 1950s to the late 1960s, almost as a rebuke to intellectualism, had a considerable impact on many aspects of society. This movement centred on the writings of Jack Kerouac and Allen Ginsberg but included many others (Norman Mailer, William Burroughs, Gregory Corso, Lawrence Ferlinghetti) at its core. These were the writers who were christened by Jack Kerouac the 'Beat Generation'.

Imagine the culture, feel the energy. There was Andy Warhol's 'Factory', there was (and still is) the Chelsea Hotel and there were 'happenings', such as Claes Oldenburg's installations. Performance art productions were taking place everywhere in Manhattan.

But it was the Beat Generation that was driving innovations, about which it has been said that is was 'altogether too vigorous, too intent, too indefatigable, too curious to suit its elders ... [it seemed] occupied with the feverish production of answers ... to a single question: how are we to live?' (Holmes 1960: 34).

Kerouac (1961) stated that:

> The word 'beat' originally meant poor, down and out, dead-beat ... now ... it is being made to stretch to include people who do not sleep in subways but have a new gesture, or attitude, which I can only describe as a new more.
>
> (Kerouac 1961: 10)

Corso added to this sentiment (1961: 56), saying that it has 'a harsh unequal voice, a voice of divinity, a new voice, conqueror eater voice, parasite of the old dead voice'.

The Beat Generation was a reaction to mid-century American anxiety and paranoia (Lee 1996) and to the 'middle-class values of the "tranquillised" fifties' (Norwich 1990: 39). Out of this feeling grew a reaction which prompted Kerouac to proclaim 'woe unto those who don't realise that America must, will, is changing now' (1961: 36) and prompted Ginsberg (1956: 112) to ask the question: 'Are you going to let your emotional life be run by *Time* magazine?'

Out of this creative movement that seemed to peak in the 1960s emerged arguably some of the greatest and potentially most influential literature to be written, art created, and music composed. Kerouac wrote *On the Road*, *The Dharma Bums* and *Desolation Angels*. William Burroughs wrote *The Naked Lunch* and *The Soft Machine*. Aldous Huxley wrote *The Doors of Perception* and *Brave New World*. Andy Warhol was deeply involved in the creation of the 'pop art' movement, turning out great works of art such as *Chairman Mao*, *Electric Chair* and, in 1962, exhibiting his famous Campbell soup tin paintings. Music was made by composers as diverse as Philip Glass, Lou Reed of the Velvet Underground and Steve Reich. The culture of New York and beyond went through radical changes. Such was the significance of the Beat Generation and their product, it could be argued that they participated in – indeed, may have been directly responsible for – developing a whole range of people's rights, including the consumer rights movement, the anti-racist movement and the gay rights movement.

William S. Burroughs

William Burroughs was always on the edge of the Beat Generation movement. Anybody who has not read his novels should do so with some caution: explicit sexual references are frequent. However, they also contain what can be interpreted as patterns of radical thought. For example, in *The Soft Machine*, the novel that followed *The Naked Lunch*, Burroughs explores issues of power. Using his non-linear 'cut-up' and 'fold-in' writing styles, which form the basis of the new research method described here, Burroughs is able to create an almost-but-more-than *Finnigan's Wake* type dynamic-multiple-reality, multi-dimensional feeling of unease, disquiet, vague recognition and recall and almost-identification, that could be said to be absent in most other more formal writing structures.

A semantic analysis of Burroughs' work (Ingram 1996) reveals the influence of Korzybski's system of 'general semantics', which 'explores possible links between human language structures and the pathology of the human mind-body in society' and offers a 'radical critique of the habitual structures of Western language' (Ingram 1996: 95) that routinely imposed false realities. It is a critical point that, in his work, Burroughs sought 'to build a language in which certain falsifications inherent in all existing languages will be made incapable of formulation' (Burroughs 1978: 12), which he thought he could achieve by eliminating certain linguistic-conceptual practices. These include linearity, the use of the definite article and other polarising binary oppositions such as 'is' and 'either/or'. Burroughs claimed that the 'is' of identity 'always carries the implication of that and nothing else, and ... the assignment of permanent condition' (Ingram 1996: 95), the traditional research 'static'. Similarly, Burroughs asserted that the use of 'the' as in 'the' universe contains implications of one and only, denying another and that 'either/or' reduces phenomena to nothing more than binary opposition and should be replaced by 'and'. This is in a similar fashion to de Saussure, who regarded the linguistic sign as 'not a link between a thing and a name, [as is our usual interpretation] but [a link] between a concept and a sound pattern' (de Saussure 1979: 98). Furthermore, Burroughs introduced elements of randomness and non-linearity into the process of textual production by using 'cut-up' and 'paste-in' or 'fold-in' techniques. This process involved Burroughs cutting up the texts that he produced and also introducing further random elements from, for example, newspapers or classic novels. He would then join up the cut-ups and fold-ins in order to create the new text. In this way, Burroughs hoped to 'make explicit a psycho-sensory process that is going on all the time anyway' (Burroughs 1978: 4). He added that writing is normally 'confined in the sequential representational straightjacket ... a form ... far removed from the actual facts of human perception and consciousness' (Burroughs 1985: 65). Life is a cut-up, he said, full of random interjections. His writing aimed to 'exorcise habitual conditioned responses, to project one's very nervous system onto some external plane (the writing machine)' (Lyndenberg 1987: 54). By using such a process, Burroughs achieves a disturbing and anxiety-provoking level of unease and vague feelings of familiarity, an awareness of different or multiple realities or at least an alteration in those realities, a sense of space/time movement, a flashback/forward, an involuntary memory, an escape from the formal and accepted structure of language and the restrictions of subjective conditioning, out of any fixed self-image perception. New connections, juxtapositions and infinite associations may be created. The word becomes an object detached from the author, the context and its signifying function; a construct that complements later thoughts on inter-textuality related by Kristeva (1982). As a result, Burroughs stated, 'one's range of vision consequently expands' (Burroughs 1978: 4).

The 'research' method emerges

Informally, Burroughs produced his first cut-up text almost by accident as he was editing and re-editing *The Naked Lunch*. However, it was not until he was working with the artist Brion Gysin some years later that he discovered that during the production of a collage he had accidentally cut through several layers of newspaper that were protecting a work surface. The resultant cut-up, attributed to Brion Gysin, was a montage of words from the *Paris Herald Tribune*, the *Observer*, the *Daily Mail* and advertisements from *Life* magazine, that was created in September 1959 and subsequently published along with other examples in *Minutes to Go* (Beiles *et al.* 1968):

The cut-up releases the text from its binding, from its author, even from its conventional signifying function, it also enables the text to regenerate.

(Lyndenberg 1987: 49)

What I am going to do is to describe a potential new method of inquiry and give an example of its use. Unlike any other method that has been applied in healthcare practice, this is not based on any other previous method, nor does it draw inspiration from any other orthodox method or research tradition. Rather, it is inspired by the work of arguably the greatest American writer of the twentieth century, William S. Burroughs, and the text construction techniques that he employed in writing such modern classics as *The Naked Lunch*, *The Soft Machine* and *Cities of the Red Night*. As stated earlier, the method is influenced by ideas that have been mirrored by general semantics and also has a more informal theoretical foundation in the work of the postmodernists and in the deconstruction genre. These are typified by, for example, Korzybski, de Saussure and Derrida. They create something akin, perhaps, to Kristeva's third party, or an emergent version of the apocalypse (Kristeva 1982). More directly, they are an acknowledgement of the postmodernist view of 'the plural nature of reality ... and the partial nature of any representation of reality that arises from any form of writing/speaking that attempts to explore, describe or explain that reality' (Cheek 2000: 5).

In order to construct a cut-up and the resultant dynamic and individual effects, perceptions and interpretations, standard text is taken and subjected to any one of a number of essentially very similar text-manipulation techniques. A computerised cut-up program, which, in the tradition of Burroughs, requires no direct/conscious text manipulation, is one option. Such a program 'deconstructs' and edits the text in a seemingly chaotic but predetermined way and produces new structures, forms and manifestations of reality, as interpreted and experienced by the reader/participant. Alternatively, a text can be physically cut up with a pair of scissors or a sharp knife either vertically, horizontally or at an angle, randomly or according to a predetermined formula (it is your choice). Thus, the researcher can take a patient or client-care scenario, pathography vignette or similar material, and re-arrange it by juxtaposing pieces of text either randomly or whilst looking for new associations and/or patterns to emerge. Additional related or perhaps non-related material (in the form of any kind of text) can also be 'folded in'. What emerges from this process is what might more formally be called the research 'results', which should not be formally analysed beyond the experience of perceiving the work. Indeed, it is critical that the emergent text is confronted at a subconscious, rather than a conscious level, if such a thing is possible. Rather than trying to understand the emergent text, the goal should be to experience it. What is achieved by using such methods is probably similar to what Burroughs aimed for in his own work, which was:

> A mutation in consciousness, [which] will occur spontaneously once certain pressures now in operation are removed. I feel that the principal instrument of monopoly and control that prevents the expansion of consciousness is the word lines controlling thought, feeling and apparent sensory impressions of the human host ... in other words, man must get away from verbal forms to attain the consciousness which is there to be perceived.
>
> (Burroughs 1978: 8)

The story of Tracey

In the following example, a computerised cut-up program has been used to manipulate the story of Tracey as it was first related by Boykin and Schoenhofer in 1991. The original text is presented first, followed by the cut-up version produced by the computer program. This second version has been slightly edited for ease of reading – beyond this no other changes have been made. Try to read the text out loud or, even better, get somebody to read it to you and just listen. Although the original text is moving and revealing in its own way, the cut-up reveals new patterns, manifestations, relationships and experiences – new appreciations of reality. As stated earlier, no attempt is or should be made to analyse the new version, as it should not really be viewed 'in terms of process and product. The experience of participating with the art creates moments anew, and the work lives for each person in a unique and special way' (Boykin *et al.* 1994: 10).

> I listened to the change of shift report and remember the strange feeling in the pit of my stomach when the evening nurse reviewed Tracey's lab tests. Tall, strawberry blond and freckle faced, Tracey was struggling with the everyday problems of adolescence and fighting a losing battle against leukemia. Tracey rarely had visitors. As I talked to Tracey that night I felt resentment from her towards her mother and experienced a sense of urgency that her mother be with her. With Tracey's permission I called her mother and told her that Tracey needed her that night. I learned that Tracey's mother was a single mother with two other small children and that she lived several hours from the hospital. When she arrived, distance and silence prevailed. With encouragement, the mother sat close to Tracey and I sat on the other side stroking Tracey's arm. I left the room to make my rounds and upon return found Tracey's mother still sitting on the edge of the bed fighting to stay awake. I gently asked Tracey if we could lie on the bed with her. She nodded. The three of us lay there and then I left the room. Later, when I returned I

found Tracey wrapped in her mothers arms. Her mother's eyes met mine as she whispered she's gone. And then she said please don't take her yet. I left the room and closed the door quietly behind me. It was just after 6 o'clock when I slipped back into the room just as the early morning light was coming through the window. I reached out and touched Tracey's mothers arm. She raised her tear-streaked face to look at me. It's time I said and waited. When she was ready I helped her off the bed and held her in my arms for a few moments. We cried together. Thank you nurse she said as she looked into my eyes and pressed my hand between hers. Then she turned and walked away.

(Boykin and Schoenhofer 1991)

The cut-up version

And I listened.

I, mother, nurse.

I sat on the edge of the bed fighting to stay awake and held her in my arms for a few moments.

We cried together. Thank you nurse she said, please don't take her yet.

I reached out and touched Tracey's mothers arm. She raised her tear-streaked face to look at me. It's time I said and waited.

Distance and silence prevailed.

We cried together. Thank you nurse she whispered, she's gone.

And then she said please don't take her yet,

I left the room.

Later, when I returned I found Tracey wrapped in her mothers arms.

Her eyes met mine. As she pressed my hand between hers.

I left the room and closed the door quietly behind me.

I reached out and touched Tracey's mothers arm.

She raised her tear-streaked face to look at me.

It's time I said and waited.

When she was ready I helped her off the bed and held her in my arms for a few moments.

We cried together.

Thank you nurse she said as she looked into my eyes.

Tall, strawberry blond and freckle faced,

Tracey rarely had visitors.

I left the room.

With encouragement, the mother sat close to Tracey that night.

I felt resentment.

She nodded.

The three of us lay there and then I left the room just as the early morning light was coming through the window.

I reached out and touched Tracey's mothers arm.

She raised her tear-streaked face to look at me. It's time I said and waited.
When she was ready I helped her off the bed.
We cried together.
Then she turned and silence prevailed.
With encouragement, the mother sat close to Tracey.
Tracey needed her that night.
It's time I said and waited.
Tall, strawberry blond and freckle faced,
Tracey was struggling with the everyday problems of adolescence and fighting a losing battle against leukemia.
Tracey rarely had visitors.
She raised her tear-streaked face to look at me.
It's time I said and waited.
I left the room.
Later, when I returned I found Tracey wrapped in her mother's arms.
Her mother's eyes met mine as she whispered she's gone.
She said please don't take her yet.
I left the room and closed the door quietly behind me.
It was just after 6 o'clock when I returned,
I found Tracey wrapped in her mother's arms.
Her eyes met mine as she whispered she's gone. She whispered she's gone.
And then she said please don't take her yet.
I left the room.
It was just after 6 o'clock when I returned.
I found Tracey wrapped in her mother's arms.
Her mother's eyes met mine as she whispered she's gone.
And then she whispered she's gone.
Tracey's mother was a single mother.
When she was ready I helped her off the bed.
I called her mother and experienced a sense of urgency that her mother …
I experienced a sense of urgency that her mother …
that her mother be with her.
She nodded.
The three of us lay there and then I left the room just as the early morning light was coming through the window.
I reached out and touched Tracey's mothers arm.
She raised her tear-streaked face to look at me.
It's time I said and waited.
When she was ready I helped her off the bed.
She nodded.
The three of us lay there and then I left the room just as the early morning light was coming through the window.
I reached out and touched Tracey's mothers arm.
She raised her tear-streaked face to look at me.

It's time I said and waited.
When she was ready I helped her off the bed and held her in my arms for a
few moments.
We cried together.
Thank you nurse she said please don't take her yet
It's time I said and waited.
Then she turned ...
Tracey's light waited.
Strawberry Tracey.
I,
She,
Nurse,
Tracey.
Hospital.
Tracey's leukemia.
Tracey needed her that ...
Tracey needed her that night.
It's time I said and waited.
We cried together.
Thank you nurse she said.
Her mother's eyes met mine.
We cried together.
And she whispered she's gone.
And then she whispered she's gone.
She turned.
Tall, strawberry blond and freckle faced,
Her eyes met mine as she whispered she's gone. She whispered she's gone.
When she was ready I helped her off the bed.
I reached out and touched Tracey's mother's arm.
She raised her tear-streaked face to look at me.
Tall, strawberry blond and freckle faced.
Her eyes met mine and then she whispered she's gone.
She turned ...

In conclusion

I hope that what I have achieved is the same as that which Burroughs aimed
for in his own work:

> A mutation in consciousness, [which] will occur spontaneously once
> certain pressures now in operation are removed. I feel that the principal
> instrument of monopoly and control that prevents the expansion of
> consciousness is the word lines controlling thought, feeling and appar-
> ent sensory impressions of the human host ... in other words, man

must get away from verbal forms to attain the consciousness which is there to be perceived.

(Burroughs 1978: 50)

However, as I was socialised into the orthodox research tradition, I began to realise that I – perhaps or even probably like so many others – was and still probably am attached 'to traditional and already accepted concepts and paradigms [that] may also overwhelm new evidence presenting a different view ... there is considerable resistance to change' (Mulhall 1995: 580), a situation that results in considerable unease when confronted with material such as that presented here. As I have played with some of the ideas presented here, over the past ten years or so, in private and in presentations and workshops in the United Kingdom and around the world, I have encountered various reactions, ranging from a possible 'resistance to change' incredulity to profound almost physically felt time-slip experiences, and I would expect the same kind of reactions to this chapter. All I ask, however, is that readers consider the above construction as an experimental possibility that just might, only might, provide an opportunity to experience these new perspectives, Mulhall's 'different view'; that just might, only might, contribute to the spectrum of methods that enable us to catch a glimpse of another's view, to 'grasp and sense the lived experience of ... clients, to enter into the world their clients inhabit' (Streubert and Carpenter 1999: 4). If you have a spare moment or two, find a piece of text; it may be a newspaper news report, your diary, a textbook or work of fiction. Photocopy it. Cut it up with a pair of scissors. See what happens. You may be surprised.

Acknowledgments

Especially to Matthew Jack, James and Anna and to all those who have given me the courage to experiment, particularly Brian, Steve Dean, Frances and Bear (Tom Cox).

References

Beiles, S., Burroughs, W. S., Corso, G. and Gysin, B. (1968) *Minutes to Go*, San Francisco: City Lights.

Boykin, A., Parker, M. E. and Schoenhofer, S. O. (1994) 'Aesthetic knowing grounded in an explicit conception of nursing', *Nursing Science Quarterly*, 7, 4: 158–61.

Boykin, A. and Schoenhofer, S. O. (1991) 'Story as link between nursing practice, ontology, epistemology', *Image: The Journal of Nursing Scholarship*, 23, 4, 245–48.

Burroughs, W. S. (1978) *The Third Mind*, New York: Viking.

Burroughs, W. S. (1985) 'The fall of Art', in *The Adding Machine: Collected Essays*, London: John Calder.

Cheek, J. (2000) *Postmodern and Poststructural Approaches to Nursing Research*, London: Sage Publications.

Corso, G. (1961) 'Variations on a generation', in Parkinson, T., ed., *A Casebook on the Beat Generation*, New York: Thomas Y. Crowell.

de Saussure, F. (1979) *Course in General Semantics*, London: Duckworth.

Ginsberg, A. (1956) 'America', in *Howl and Other Poems*, San Francisco: City Lights Books.

Holmes, J. C. (1960) 'The philosophy of the Beat Generation', in Krim, S., ed., *The Beats*, Connecticut: Fawcett.

Ingram, D. (1996) 'William Burroughs and language', in Lee, A. R., ed., *The Beat Generation Writers*, London: Pluto Press.

Kerouac, J. (1961) 'The origins of the Beat Generation', in Parkinson, T., ed., *A Casebook on the Beat Generation*, New York: Thomas Y. Crowell.

Kristeva, J. (1982) *Powers of Horror: An Essay on Abjection*, New York: Columbia University Press.

Lee, A. R. (1996) 'Introduction', in Lee, A. R., ed., *The Beat Generation Writers*, London: Pluto Press.

Lyndenberg, R. (1987) 'Word cultures: Radical theory and practice', in *William S. Burroughs' Fiction*, Urbana: University of Illinois Press.

Lyotard, J. (1984) *The Postmodern Condition: A Report on Knowledge*, Minneapolis: University of Minnesota Press.

Mulhall, A. (1995) 'Nursing research: what difference does it make?', *Journal of Advanced Nursing*, 21, 3: 576–83.

Norwich, J. J., ed., (1990) *The Oxford Illustrated Encyclopaedia of The Arts*, Oxford: Oxford University Press.

Streubert, H. J. and Carpenter, D. R. (1999) *Qualitative Research in Nursing: Advancing the Humanistic Imperative*, Philadelphia: Lippincott.

Chapter 8

Historiography, illness and the interpretation of fiction

Christopher Maggs

At the centre of this paper is an early Victorian clerk, Mr Chuffey, a character devised by Charles Dickens in *Martin Chuzzlewit* (Dickens [1844] 1999) to enable a murder to be exposed and for good to prevail. He enters the novel in Chapter 11 as a comic and pathetic figure in contrast to another of the central characters, Pecksniff, who is comic and duplicitous. Chuffey about 'Twenty years ago or so he went and took a fever' (Dickens [1844] 1999: 178). At a critical point in the novel, he reveals facts surrounding the death of his employer, which exonerates the would-be murderer of killing his own father. As we shall see, his employer was not murdered but died of natural causes, although Chuffey's intervention leads on to the exposure of a real murder, that of the business accomplice of his late master's son. Typical Dickensian twists and turns combine to show the moral differences between American and English culture of the day.

This paper explores historical method – historiography – and its rigour through an analysis of the representation of one man's illness and its meaning in the context of the author's literary, political and societal intent. Thus it fits with the overall aim of this volume – the exploration of new methodologies to enlighten our understanding of health and social care issues. It uses a case study approach in which a fictional depiction of a Victorian clerk, who appears to have some disability, is discussed in order to gain insights into the lives of real clerks in that period and what might be the outcome of a man who has suffered some kind of cerebral vascular accident (stroke). If asked why, my response would be that we have a fascination as historians with the Victorian era because, of all historical epochs, it has most influence on and resonance with our own. The world of work, for example, created through industrialism, finds its consequences in our own times; the importance of providing for old age, now through personal/state pensions, then through 'loyalty', is an immediate concern, and the continuing fallout from 'Thatcherism' dogs our views of personal versus community/state responsibility.

The paper starts by looking at the history of historiography and the ways in which approaches to history have changed over time. A brief review of medical history or the history of medicine follows, which allows the scene to be set for an exploration of Mr Chuffey's illness and the historical analysis. The final section returns to the contribution historiography can make to our development of new methodologies in the humanities.

On the history of historiography

In his book *The Whig Interpretation of History* (Butterfield 1931), Butterfield presents an argument that the past – history – must fit with the present; that, as Cooter puts it about the historiography of phrenology, 'nothing can be true in the past which conflicts with what is known in the present' (Cooter 1984: 16). Thus historians are free to make judgements about the past and to show it as false or wrong because, it is argued, they have value-free or neutral knowledge gained by a scientific approach to understanding. This positivist ideological stance seeks to identify certain types of knowledge as 'incorrect (because of their having unquantitative human, social or metaphysical dimensions) in order to establish the impression of other bodies of knowledge as value-transcendent touchstones of truth' (Cooter 1984: 18).

Such a perspective has had challenges and revisions, particularly since the development of social history as a discipline. For example, Brian Abel-Smith sought to defend the changes proposed by himself and other key policy informers and makers in the National Health Service in the 1960s, having reviewed its first decade of existence. Abel-Smith did so in part by looking at nursing, its organisation and role, through his historical account of the development of the profession. Here, Abel-Smith could look back from the vantage point of 1960, when nursing was about to be transformed, to a period when its function could be described as little more than 'a specialised form of charring' (cited in Maggs 1980: 4). These early antecedents could then be contrasted with the educated, skilled and organised nurses needed by the 'new' NHS for the 1960s and 1970s. In so doing, Abel-Smith only slightly revised the Whig approach and completely failed to note, for instance, any understanding of why individual women might enter the occupation, whether in the 1890s or the 1960s.

In the history of medicine, as Brieger notes, significant change has taken place in the past 30 years, led by the work of George Rosen. Citing Rosen (Rosen 1967), Brieger writes that:

> A shift in the angle of vision not infrequently reveals new facets of a subject, and this has happened to the history of medicine. By taking the social character of medicine as a point of departure, the history of medicine becomes the history of human societies and their efforts to deal with problems of health and disease.
>
> (Brieger 1993: 25)

As I have written elsewhere (Maggs 2002: 12), historical accounts are, by their very nature, selective and owe as much to the author's judgements as to their relative importance. This also includes the author's own history and context. Lytton Strachey (Strachey 1931) wrote that 'facts relating to the past, when they are collected without art, are compilations; and compilations, no doubt, may be useful; but they are no more History than butter, eggs, salt and herbs are an omelette' (cited in Maggs 2002: 12). Much of revisionist history remains replete with positivist values and much lacks the unquantitative understanding that comprises the humanness of the subjects and the historians.

Just as the rise of social history has freed historians from the chains of positivism and doxology (the formulaic praise of a 'great one'), so the history of medicine has discovered 'those who suffered ... the legion of workers, men and women, who for so long waged the daily battle against the ravages of ill health, but who, in the histories of medicine, were as anonymous as their counterparts in society had been in the general histories' (Brieger 1993: 27). This more confident history of medicine community has added new skills for understanding to its repertoire, including the humanities, anthropology, literary criticism and cultural studies (Brieger 1993: 27–8).

Although those historians more in tune with doxology have also tended to use several sources – personal papers of 'great men', their reminiscences, state or organisation documents – the increasing utilisation of other disciplines in constructing the new history of medicine, as with social history itself, necessitates a more painstaking approach to historical sources. Today, historians will use personal testimony and oral history, documentary analysis, economic and other statistical data in constructing an account. However, the principle challenge in such cases is to understand and make a decision about the relative weighting each kind of source merits. For example, are the data about coal production set out in tonnes per year per colliery of the same order as the oral testimony of an individual miner describing his experience of working a 12-hour shift to produce sufficient coal to earn a bonus? Is the document produced by the Ministerial Department for internal use of the same order as a report in Hansard?

Acknowledging that this matters is important to rigorous historical investigation, although rather than weigh each piece of evidence against another or some neutral arbitrary measure, it might be more helpful to maintain a general scepticism about all evidence, no matter the source. That would require corroboration rather than some exercise in measurement of value or merit.

The story of Mr Chuffey

Given his crucial role in helping to acquit the villain of patricide only to expose the foul murder of the villain's business partner, it is surprising that Mr Chuffey, Mr Pecksniff's clerk, gets no attention in writings on Charles Dickens' *Martin Chuzzlewit* (Dickens [1844] 1999). Perhaps even more so, since the character was played as recently as 1994 on the London stage by John Mills. It is my contention, however, that Dickens needed not just the character of the faithful clerk, but such a character who was also ill, and ill with a specific condition, in order to be able to end his story successfully.

First, a résumé of the plot is needed, to set the scene and to begin the process of historical analysis, if only such an endeavour were possible! The purpose of the novel was to argue that English culture and society excelled over those of the USA – which Dickens had recently visited – in a number of ways, not least in its use of language and social mores. Dickens uses the device of selfishness to explore this idea, and each of the principal characters, including the erstwhile 'hero', comes out badly. The 'hero', Martin Chuzzlewit, goes to America as a result of disappointment – personal and professional – in England, only to discover criminality, fraud, deception and degradation there. Escaping ignominiously, he returns to England to find that he has a potential career as an architect. His earlier preparation for that career has been at the hands of Mr Pecksniff, who takes in pupils at exorbitant charges but has never qualified nor practised in that capacity. Martin's cousin, Jonas Chuzzlewit, buys some poison from a minor character, the doctor/assistant Lewsome, putting it in a place he knows his father will find and eat it. He is seen hiding the doctored paste by Mr Chuffey, the aged and loyal, sick and deformed clerk. The older Mr Chuzzlewit falls to the floor in a faint and is carried upstairs to bed. Jonas believes he has killed his father but in fact, as Chuffey discovers, the old man is dying of probably a stroke or heart attack. Jonas marries one of Pecksniff's daughters, whom he does not love and whom, as Emily Brontë's Heathcliff does to his 'surrogate wife', he sets out to destroy for her love of him. Jonas, becoming a bit of a fraud, ends up killing his partner, Tiggs Macauley, in a series of acts reminiscent and worthy of *Macbeth*. In a scene that resembles a later Hercule Poirot dénouement, Jonas is confronted about a series of events by, including others, a corrupt 'detective' who has 'gone underground' to find evidence to convict Jonas of murder, but murder not of Anthony Chuzzlewit but of Tiggs! Mr Chuffey exonerates Jonas from patricide, although he reveals that he knows that Jonas had attempted Anthony Chuzzlewit's murder. Faced with his guilt for the death of Tiggs, Jonas kills himself and, although no one comes out of it unblemished, the best people at least seem less ambiguous about right and wrong than those who do not.

Commentators see in the novel Dickens trying to suggest that even if everyone is less than honest, it is in America that this manifests itself in the public as opposed to the private domain. His own experiences in that country had clearly made him convinced that England was morally superior. However, as Patricia Ingham, in the 'Introduction' to the Penguin Classics edition, says:

> Overall the country to which Chuzzlewit and Tapley return retrospectively casts a better light on America where at least victims know what they are up against ... What he [Dickens] appears inadvertently to have done is explore the intertwining of moral sensibility and brutality, and an incompatibility between virtue and power that creates a nightmare not in America but in England.
>
> (Ingham 1999: xxv)

But what of Chuffey, how 'real' was he? We first hear that he has had a breakdown of some sort 20 years before, seems to have spent that time counting to several million before he became 'better' and spends most of his time 'hidden' or in the dark area beside the fire. This is a typically 'early' Dickensian device, as Page (1984) argues. In Page's view, the novel lacks a central drama, as much of what happens takes place on the periphery. Chuffey is later said to have a physical weakness in his arm and known to be weak of mind by the nurse employed to look after him.

Mr Chuffey appears in Chapter 11. Jonas has invited the two unmarried Pecksniff daughters to his family home. Called into the room, Chuffey enters:

> A little blear-eyed, weazen-faced, ancient man came creeping out. He was of remote fashion, and dusty, like the rest of the furniture; he was dressed in a decayed suit of black; with breeches garnished at the knees with rusty wisps of ribbon, the very paupers of shoe-strings; on the lower portion of his spindly legs were dingy worsted stockings of the same colour. He looked as if he had been put away and forgotten half a century before, and somebody had just found him in a lumber-closet.
>
> (Dickens [1844] 1999: 177)

His gait is described as he enters the room as 'slowly creeping'. His 'dim faculties became conscious of the presence of strangers, and those strangers ladies, he rose again (from the chair), apparently intending to make a bow' (Dickens [1844] 1999: 177). However, he is too feeble and sinks back down into the chair, where he breathes 'on his shrivelled hands to warm them, remained with his poor blue nose immovable above his plate, looking at nothing, with eyes that saw nothing, and a face that meant nothing. Nothing else' (*ibid*. p. 177). The guests ask if he is deaf or blind and, when asked, are told that he is neither. 'What is he then?' (*ibid*. p. 178) comes the question.

Jonas explains that 'he's precious old, for one thing; and I an't best pleased with him for that for I think my father must have caught it off him' (*ibid*. p. 178). Jonas elaborates:

> Why, you see ... he's been addling his old brains with figures and book-keeping all his life; and twenty years ago or so he went and took a fever. All that time he was out of his head (which was three weeks) he never left off casting up; and he got to so many million at last that I don't believe he's ever been quite right since. We don't do much business now though, and he an't a bad clerk.
>
> (Dickens [1844] 1999: 178)

During the meal, it becomes apparent that Mr Chuffey has difficulty in chewing his food, 'but the mutton being tough, and his gums weak, he quickly verified the statement relative to his choking propensities, and underwent so much in his attempts to dine that Mr Jonas was infinitely amused' (*ibid*. p. 179). Jonas knows that 'he always chokes himself if it an't broth' and had deliberately not had broth just to see the old man choke and to amuse himself and his guests! In the end, Mr Chuffey, making no progress at all with the mutton, is told to just 'peg away at his bread' (*ibid*. p. 179). In an aside with dramatic prescience, Jonas tells the Pecksniff daughters that 'he was afraid one of these fine days, Chuffey would be the death of him' (*ibid*. p. 179).

A little later, old Anthony Chuzzlewit proudly goes to tell his clerk how Jonas is following in his footsteps, as a duplicitous businessman, whose precept was 'do other men, for they would do you' (*ibid*. p. 180). Mr Chuffey 'rubbed his hands, nodded his palsied head, winked his watery eyes and cried in whistling tones, Good! Good!' (*ibid*. p. 180). However, even though Chuffey seemed to share these sentiments, even old Anthony knew that if anyone had a remaining spark of humanity left, it was 'yet lingering at the bottom of the worn-out cask, called Chuffey' (*ibid*. p. 181).

It is in Chapter 18 that the death of Anthony Chuzzlewit is portrayed and where we learn that Chuffey has a 'palsied arm' (*ibid*. p. 290). Discussing the possibility of Jonas marrying one of Pecksniff's daughters, Charity, Anthony Chuzzlewit mulls over death, which Pecksniff would like to happen relatively soon in Chuzzlewit's case so that his daughter will be well taken care of when Jonas inherits. Anthony snarls that he has years of life left and really it should be Chuffey who should be expiring, 'why, look at him, pointing to his feeble clerk. Death has no right to leave him standing, and to mow me down' (*ibid*. p. 294).

Anthony Chuzzlewit's death takes place over one night. We see him, Jonas, Pecksniff and Chuffey in the parlour, discussing money and marriage in their corrupt fashion. But Chuzzlewit seems more tired than usual and soon falls asleep besides the fire, a place often taken by Chuffey himself. A little later, there comes an extraordinary noise, 'upon my word, Mr Jonas, that is a very extraordinary clock, said Pecksniff. It would have been, if it had made the noise which startled them; but another kind of time-piece was fast running down, and from that the sound proceeded' (*ibid*. p. 296). Anthony is taken up to his bed, where the doctor bleeds him, but to no great avail. Next morning, he is helped downstairs, dressed by Chuffey, and enters the parlour, almost frightening the life out of Jonas, who is worried that his deed will be found out. Anthony tries to speak to Jonas and Pecksniff but the words 'were such as man had never heard. And this was the most fearful circumstance of all, to see him standing there, gabbling in an unearthly tongue' (*ibid*. p. 298). Despite Chuffey's assertion that the old man was 'better now', he dies peacefully in his chair in front of the window a little later (*ibid*. p. 299).

Mr Chuffey makes his final appearance in Chapter 51 when young Martin Chuzzlewit confronts Jonas about Anthony's death. Mr Chuffey intervenes to explain that Jonas did not actually poison his father, because he and Anthony knew about the doctored paste and Anthony had not taken any of it. On his deathbed, Anthony Chuzzlewit had implored his clerk not to denounce his son: 'Spare him, Cuff! I promised him I would. I've tried to do it. He's his only son' (*ibid*. p. 734). As he explained in the scene where Jonas is finally confronted with his crime, Chuffey had agreed because 'We were at school together, he and I. I couldn't turn against his son, you know – his only son, Mr Chuzzlewit!' (*ibid*. p. 731).

The Victorian clerk

Mr Chuffey's story can be re-presented through textual analysis of the novel *Martin Chuzzlewit*. However, as we shall show, its historical import needs more contextualisation and we do this through a brief exploration of the world of the Victorian clerk, using non-literary sources.

The Victorian clerk in the counting house or commercial or legal firm often appears in Dickens' work, usually as a caricature (see Bob Cratchit in *A Christmas Carol*, or Uriah Heep in *David Copperfield*, for example). Data about the precise number of clerks before 1861 are hard to corroborate. However, in 1861 there were just under 100,000 men employed mainly in London and the large manufacturing cities of Leeds, Manchester and Liverpool, as clerks of one kind or another (Holcombe 1973: 210). Most were employed, at least until after Dickens' death in 1870, in small establishments, usually family firms, or small-scale partnerships (*ibid*. p. 142). Underneath the clerks were premium-paying apprentices, learning the trade at no cost to the employer. According to Holcombe, many clerks came from the middle class or at least that section of society that could read, write and add up (*ibid*. p. 142). As Chuffey himself notes, he and old Anthony Chuzzlewit were at school together: 'we learnt Tare and Tret [rules for calculating net weight] together, at school. I took him down once, six boys in the arithmetic class. God forgive me! Had I the heart to take him down!' (Dickens [1844] 1999: 307).

When Dickens published *Martin Chuzzlewit*, *Pitman's Shorthand* had been published for about five years, although it was to be some ten years more before there was any evidence that it was being used routinely in commerce (Holcombe 1973: 143). At the time of publication of *Martin Chuzzlewit*, literacy levels were generally low and Holcombe suggests therefore that the clerk might be regarded as a skilled worker and 'In the small family concerns ... there was "an almost feudal relationship" between clerks and their employers. The clerk was more a family servant than a waged labourer' (Holcombe 1973: 149). It was common for clerks to 'live in' and to share the family table, as did Mr Chuffey.

Whilst universal education did not come for several decades, spelling the demise of the skilled clerical worker, all such workers faced a constant threat – a sword of Damocles which was the possibility of losing their job for one reason or another, bankruptcy, death of the employer, and so on. If that happened, especially after a certain age, the prospects for further employment were almost non-existent. Like many workers at the lower end of the middle classes, as indeed with the employers and their families, the prospect of falling into the abyss of poverty and destitution was a constant. This was the era, the 1840s, which formed the basis for Engel's polemic, *The Condition of the Working Class in England*, the time of the 'most catastrophic economic slump of the nineteenth century, that of 1841–2' (Hobsbawm in Engels [1892] 1974: 14) and the Irish Famine.

Mr Chuffey's illness

Dickens presents us with a portrait, really a partial portrait, of the Victorian clerk. He wrote of others but Mr Chuffey stands out for two reasons. First, he is portrayed not just as a clerk but one who has been ill and yet remains in employment. Second, he is crucial to the denouncing of a murderer. It is the first reason that concerns us here. What might Mr Chuffey have suffered from and does Dickens' portrait tell us anything about that illness?

Mr Chuffey had, some twenty years before, suffered a fever, lasting about three weeks, during which he counted and counted repetitively, as though he were at work at his ledgers. His recovery left him able to walk but feebly and to speak but he remains silent (although we have no inkling of his previous mode) unless addressed first by his employer. (He only answers others or becomes spontaneous much later in the story when the finale approaches.) He has a palsied arm, watery eyes that often appear lifeless, thin, cold hands that he constantly tries to warm by blowing on them, a blue nose, and difficulty in eating and swallowing. He spends much of his time sitting in the shadows beside the fire but, when required, is still able to do his job well. And, at times, he can become quite excitable, 'Aye, aye!, cried the old man, brightening up as before, when this was communicated to him in the same voice; quite right, quite right. He's your own son, Mr Chuzzlewit! Bless him for a sharp lad! Bless him, bless him!' (Dickens [1844] 1999: 179).

The novel was published in its entirety in 1844, and we may, with licence, assume that the events therein take place around that time rather than much earlier and are certainly not futuristic.

It is inappropriate to attempt a diagnosis at such a remove – not just temporal but because the character is, after all, a fictional construct. Some historians of medicine have attempted a retrospective diagnosis of, usually, great men or women, with variable degrees of success. Perhaps the best has been to show that George III suffered from porphyria and not 'madness', whilst there is continued speculation over the plight of Victorian women such as Florence Nightingale. However, it might be possible to set Mr Chuffey's illness within some sort of diagnostic framework. If it matches that framework, we could feel that Dickens had portrayed not merely the character of the Victorian clerk but one suffering from the after-effects of a particular illness or disease.

So far as we can understand, Mr Chuffey is Anthony Chuzzlewit's contemporary – they were at school together – and so he must be close to his age, which, in his 'delirium', Chuffey counts to be 'three score and ten ... ought and carry seven' (Dickens [1844] 1999: 307). Chuffey had thus suffered his 'fever' at about 57 years of age, perhaps a little older. He is described as thin, and so obesity as a causative factor might be ruled out. According to Benjamin Rush (1745–1813), cited by Wilson (1993: 400), 'fever was preceded by debility that caused excitability to accumulate, making the body susceptible to such pathogens as contagia, miasma, or injury, any of which could bring about an irregular action of the arterial system'. Rush was, according to Wilson (Wilson 1993: 400) 'the most influential medical teacher in America and his advocacy of the vigorous use of calomel and bloodletting was widely accepted by American physicians in the early nineteenth century'. Dickens, like Florence Nightingale, was a miasmist in spirit, as his novels show. The degradation of parts of London, he wrote, was responsible for the ill health and poverty found there, demonstrated by the bad air and over-reaching contagion. It was also true that Dickens, as others, saw that time as an epoch of momentous proportions, bringing with it the new diseases of civilisation, brought about by 'the frantic acceleration in the pace of living, the mad crush of humanity in the city of dreadful night, the power of the money demon and the cash nexus, the deluge of information and business ... and all the demands they were laying upon stamina' (Porter 1993: 593).

Mr Chuffey's breakdown, whether physical or mental or both, fits with the indications of some kind of brain haemorrhage or, as contemporaries might have described it, apoplexy. If the cause was a clot rather than a bleed, physicians believed that recovery was likely to be better, although the underlying pathology was little understood. A 1976 edition of a medical textbook suggests that the stereotype candidate for apoplexy, 'stout build, a short neck, and florid complexion, is now generally discredited' (Thomson 1976: 56).

Problems with speech and, in particular, swallowing are now known to be problems associated with stroke or cerebral vascular accident. Mr Chuffey's difficulties at mealtimes could be the result of poor teeth; however, his real problem is that, even if he can chew food, he gets paroxysms of choking when trying to swallow anything other than 'broth'.

However, without a full description of the original event, diagnosis can be at best be tentative, at worse, wrong. What we do know is that, whatever the precipitating cause, the patient, Mr Chuffey, is left with residual disablement, both physical and mental, but not sufficiently disabling to prevent him from working, even in the limited capacity that the firm required, nor from recalling with great accuracy events in the past.

Mr Chuffey, infirm Victorian clerk

It was important for the plot that Mr Chuffey was infirm, because he could then be ignored. Had he been able-bodied, Chuffey would have been portrayed going about his work, as other clerks are in Dickens' canon. Jonas would have needed to avoid him more in his plans to do away with his father. As it was, Mr Chuffey could be safely ignored, brought out of the shadows only for amusement or to be mocked by Jonas.

Concluding remarks

Dickens' ability to commentate on contemporary society is generally acknowledged, even where he steps over into composite and caricature. However, it is important to note that in his novels, he is describing characters not creating accurate portraits of actual individuals – it is, after all, fiction. Why, then, might an historian want to use Dickens' portrayals as a source for historical scholarship? One reason might be that the character is so strongly pictured that it comes to represent the collectivity rather than the individual. To attempt to describe the entirety of Victorian clerks, even if narrowed down to those working in small family businesses, might leave us with bare statements and facts and with little humanness. The historian therefore turns to literature like this for a composite portrait. In order to feel comfortable with that decision, the historian must be sure that the portrait is as accurate as possible. Thus, we need to seek out the raw data from whichever source we can, and make judgements about consistency and reliability for the fictional characterisation.

In the case of *Martin Chuzzlewit*, Dickens does not appear to be making a crusading comment – at least, insofar as Victorian clerks are concerned.

He is making a point about contemporary nurses, through his satire of Sarah Gamp and Betsy Prig, but not about the clerk, Mr Chuffey. We are left to wonder whether this means that Chuffey is less formed as a character and hence less reliable as a source, or more of a caricature because Dickens had leisure to make him so. It becomes a judgement, but one which can be informed by reading into the context, as we have outlined here.

Finally, we can ask three questions suggested by our reading of the novel and our understanding of historiography. Does Dickens give us a 'realistic' fictional account of the Victorian clerk? Yes, I think he does on this occasion and would point in evidence to his demonstration of the similarities between the two worlds of employer and clerk. Does Dickens give a 'realistic', fictional account of the working life of the Victorian clerk? No, because it is not his concern, except to note that Mr Chuffey continues to work well even though old and infirm. Third, does Dickens portray a man who has suffered from a specific illness that has left its mark on him and can we name that illness and residuum from what we are told? No, we are left with too many questions – for example, what was the actual event that confined Chuffey for three weeks? What was he like before that event? What symptoms does he exhibit that are to do with that event and which might be more to do with the general ageing process for that historical time and group?

The social historian, coming to one of the great social commentators in the nineteenth-century novel, is disappointed to find a partial picture with regard to the combined issues of the Victorian clerk and the depiction of illness and incapacity. That is not to castigate Dickens: he had not set out to write such a piece for the latter-day historian. Our attention to the application of a rigorous historical methodology leaves us without this novel for a source, but at least we have not lost our way. We have not weighed one kind of information against another; rather we have maintained our scepticism, sought corroboration and found the novel wanting. As Brody cautions, we should not look to illness as a metaphor, but look to literature for accurate 'descriptions of the plight of the sick person' (Brody 1987: 64–5). Researchers in health and social care, as this volume illustrates, need to heed this final comment for rigorous research – not weighing in the balances of probability but searching for corroboration with a sceptical lens.

Acknowledgement

My thanks go to Frances Rapport for the opportunity to contribute this chapter and to Trudi Williams, my muse.

References

Brieger, G. (1993) 'The historiography of medicine', in *Companion Encyclopedia of the History of Medicine*, London: Routledge.

Brody, H. (1987) *Stories of Sickness*, London: Yale University Press.

Butterfield, H. (1931) *The Whig Interpretation of History*, London: W.W. Norton.

Cooter, R. (1984) *The Cultural Meaning of Popular Science. Phrenology and the Organisation of Consent in Nineteenth-Century Britain*, Cambridge: Cambridge University Press.

Dickens, C. ([1844] 1999) *Martin Chuzzlewit*, London: Penguin.

Hobsbawm, E. (1974) 'Introduction', in Engels, F., *The Condition of the Working Class*, St Albans: Panther (first published 1892).

Holcombe, L. (1973) *Victorian Ladies at Work*, Newton Abbot: David and Charles.

Ingham, P. (1999) 'Introduction', in *Martin Chuzzlewit*, London: Penguin.

Maggs, C. (1980) 'Aspects of general hospital nursing 1881–1914', unpublished PhD thesis, University of Bath.

Maggs, C. (2002) 'Milestones in British nursing', in Daly, J., Speedy, S., Jackson, D. and Derbyshire, P., eds, *Contexts of Nursing: An Introduction*, Oxford: Blackwell.

Page, N (1984) *A Dickens' Companion*, London: Macmillan.

Porter, R. (1993) 'Diseases of civilisation', in *Companion Encyclopedia of the History of Medicine*, London: Routledge.

Rosen, G. (1967) 'People, disease and emotion. Some newer problems for research in medical history', *Bulletin of the History of Medicine*, 4: 5–23.

Strachey, L. (1931) *Portraits in Miniature and Other Essays*, London: Chatto & Windus.

Thomson, W. A. R. (1976) *Black's Medical Dictionary*, London: Adam & Charles Black.

Wilson, L. G. (1993) 'Fevers', in Bynum, W. F. and Porter, R., eds, *Companion Encyclopedia of the History of Medicine*, London: Routledge.

Chapter 9

Methodology and practical application of the Social Action Research model

Jennie Fleming and Dave Ward

The approach presented in this chapter – Social Action Research – illustrates a particular perspective in qualitative research methodology. In introducing Social Action Research, we will address three conceptual areas: empowerment, approaches to research (in particular participatory approaches) and self-directed groupwork (or Social Action). These are the distinctive elements that come together in practice to produce Social Action Research.

Empowerment

The Dictionary of Social Work (Thomas and Pierson 1995) suggests that there are two key elements to empowerment. The first is the way people attain collective control over their lives in order to achieve their interests. It is about what people – users, consumers, patients – actually *do*. The second is a method that practitioners might *use* to enhance power for those people lacking power. In other words, empowerment is the state of affairs that is reached, but also a methodology for working with people to achieve that state of affairs. An American writer, Staples (1990), produces a commonly used definition of empowerment, identifying three key themes that mix the two elements identified above. He states that empowerment involves the participation of people in their own empowerment, so it is something that people do for themselves. It also involves recognising and valuing the existing competences of people. Finally, empowerment involves building on both individual and collective strengths to arrive at what people can achieve when they work together. Thus, empowerment is a process by which power is developed or gained by the powerless.

In the theoretical writings on empowerment, there is strong debate surrounding the word 'gain' and its meaning. Some argue that power has to be seized (Baistow 1994; Braye and Preston-Shoot 1995); others say that gaining power can be facilitated by skilled and sensitive professionals (Mullender and Ward 1991; Breton 1994). Those arguing for the facilitation of empowerment by professionals are often accused by other sociological theorists of engaging in something which is simply another, albeit hidden, form of social control, which in the final analysis promotes professional self-interest (Baistow 1994; Page 1992). We argue here that empowerment can be achieved by skilled professionals working in partnership with people, be they patients, community members or service users. Such empowerment can offer people the chance to try out and experience new ways of influencing their life chances through the transformation of power relationships, with an emphasis on that word 'transform'.

The American black feminist activist, Audrey Lorde, offers some insight into what is meant by 'transforming' relationships. Lorde says:

> The true focus of revolutionary change is never merely the oppressive situations which we seek to escape, but that piece of the oppressor which is planted deep within each of us, and which knows only the oppressor's tactics and the oppressor's relationships.
>
> (Lorde 1984: 123)

Empowerment is about social change but also about personal change, personal change in those people who find themselves on both sides of the power relationship.

Our approach to empowerment is through action and a change process. This position is influenced by the work of both Michel Foucault (1980), the French philosopher and sociologist, and Stephen Lukes (1974). Their work highlights the possibility of moving beyond a 'zero sum' conception of empowerment. For them, empowerment is not something you either have or have not; not merely something which, for one group to have, must be taken away from another. Suzy Braye and Michael Preston-Shoot (1995) clarify the concept when they write about the need to view power not as a negative concept (as the 'zero sum' idea suggests) but as a positive one. As such, it should be used proactively by each party in an encounter to promote the party's own interests and to respond sensitively and knowledgeably to the interests of the other parties.

We view empowerment as operating at both individual and collective levels, in the sense that collective empowerment and the capacity of people to have greater control over their life chances also means transformation of people's own understanding and experience of their own power and what power means to them. In particular, it is about moving out of taken-for-granted assumptions that we cannot achieve change, to understanding and experiencing that there are possibilities for development and change. To do that involves engaging in new forms of relationships, working with others within the recognition that people always have some degree of control over their own life situations. In this way, individual and collective empowerment are closely intertwined.

Participatory approaches to research

A second area of exploration in Social Action Research relates to the research 'perspective'. To state the obvious, a basic requirement of social research is to obtain data from people. However, social scientists employ different methods of understanding social phenomena. The positivist approach works on the assumption that social phenomena can be explained scientifically, based on regularities in the data obtained. Positivists use tools such as surveys or questionnaires to gather data and, very often, numerical approaches to analysing and reporting data findings. In contrast, the interpretive tradition seeks to understand phenomena from the viewpoint of the people themselves. People's active response to social reality possesses meaning, and research involves engaging with people to discover the meaning behind the action in particular situations. A third approach is participatory research, where participatory researchers seek not only to discover meaning but to explore its properties with the people studied. Data are generated and verified with the people themselves. The research subjects become research participants, working in partnership with researchers to engage in a process of defining and interpreting data. The notion of empowerment is most closely aligned with this third approach.

Self-directed groupwork (Social Action)

The third area of consideration in Social Action Research is the 'Social Action' itself. Social Action has developed over the past 20 years out of a specific groupwork method – 'self-directed groupwork' (Mullender and Ward 1991 cf. Fleming and Ward 1999; Fleming 2000; Ward 2000). In the 1990s, Social Action evolved as a partnership among users, practitioners and academics through a range of activities: fieldwork, training, consultancy and research. Social Action is distinctive and should not be confused with the generic term 'social action', which describes activity aimed at bringing about social change (Staub-Bernisconi 1991). Social action, in this generalised sense, is not a term used much in the UK, but a very common expression for social change activity in the USA.

Initially, Social Action was influenced strongly by the ideas of Paulo Freire (1970), the Brazilian liberationist educator. In the 1980s and 1990s, as it developed, Social Action drew heavily on the thinking and writings of the disability movement (for example see Oliver 1990; Zarb 1992; Ward 1997; Morris 1998), the black activist movement (see Gilroy 1987; Ahmed 1990; Cress-Wesling 1991; Hooks 1992) and the feminist movement (see Dominelli and McLeod 1989; Hudson 1989; Langan and Day 1992). Social Action has also taken into account more recent developments in the literature on participation (see Fitzpatrick *et al.* 1999; Beresford 2000; Kemshall and Littlechild 2000; Wilson and Beresford 2000; Willow 2002). From the work of these writers it is possible to deduce a practice methodology to meet the goals of empowerment.

Specifically, Social Action seeks to distance itself from 'deficit' and 'blaming the victim' approaches to understanding people's behaviour. It opposes models based on individual pathology that have dominated social welfare. Rather, Social Action concentrates on the circumstances in which people find themselves. Individual pathologies are no substitute for serious consideration of the social condition of service users.

Central to Social Action is an understanding of the reasons why these conditions are what they are. 'Why' is the catchphrase of Social Action workers. In our experience, we have found that practice which claims to be participatory, too often jumps from the question 'what' to the question 'how', without considering the question 'why' in between. It is the question 'why' in the Social Action process that is critical, because if we ask people to define their problems and identify the things that trouble them, they will do so within the world that they already understand and within the framework of their existing understandings. If you go on to say, 'Can you think of some ideas as to what can be done to change your circumstances?', then the framework for the change ideas that they think of has already been set. It has been set within the status quo. It is only by asking the question 'why', and pursuing the question 'why', that people are able to get out of the constraints of their existing understandings to come up with new, innovatory ideas for changing their circumstances. So asking the question 'why' is the critical area of empowerment practice. Empowerment practice and Social Action practice hence focus on process rather than a preoccupation with outcome or task.

Social Action combines a set of principles, or value positions, together with a process for addressing problems and taking action for change. (For more information, see Centre of Social Action's website www.dmu.ac.uk/~dmucsa.) It is core to empowerment and to Social Action to have trust in the process. If you trust the process and follow it through in a disciplined way, then the tasks will be achieved and outcomes will emerge. Certainly, it does have to be accepted that the outcomes may not be the ones that professionals had either wanted or anticipated in the first place.

There are a number of key principles of Social Action Research. First, Social Action Research involves starting from the ideas and understanding of a range of stakeholders. This does not mean only including users or patients or consumers, but of all the stakeholders who have an interest in a particular research process. Social Action Research involves respecting and viewing positively stakeholders as 'knowers'. It involves a realisation that research, just as empowerment practice, is a process of learning, development and change, and that the researcher is a practitioner, as much as a researcher, in facilitating that process.

So what do Social Action Researchers do? They set in motion a process of participation with stakeholders. They work with stakeholders to shape agendas, make decisions and affect outcomes. They are involved in a non-hierarchical relationship with participants, recognising everybody as having an equal but different contribution to make to the research process. Social Action Researchers bring their analytical and data collection skills to bear, whilst stakeholders bring their knowledge of the area to be researched. The researcher influences the process by being part of it – that is implicit in the notion of participatory research. Data analysis and dissemination are undertaken jointly, and stakeholders are helped to act on their new knowledge and understanding. Social Action Research involves a responsibility not to leave the participants and the stakeholders high and dry at the end of the research process, having learnt a great deal but not knowing or having any ideas about what actions to take towards change. Social Action Research involves moving from understanding and knowledge into action. It is important to clarify that Social Action Research does contrast with other ideas of user-centred research, most clearly articulated by Peter Beresford who stresses user control (Beresford and Evans 1999). Social Action Research is not based on user control, but on partnership.

The second principle of Social Action Research involves a distinct methodology. Shaw (2000) makes a distinction between methodology and methods. Methods are techniques by which data are collected, for example, observations or questionnaires. Most methods, but by no means all, can be adapted to service a particular methodology. Methodology is a broader concept that takes into account theoretical and value premises and the social processes through which research is carried out. Thus, Social Action Research is a methodology, which will be set out in the next part of this chapter. However, within the Social Action Research methodology there are many methods that are familiar to researchers of all dispositions.

Finally we offer an acronym, which might act as a reminder of Social Action Research and its key characteristics. The acronym – though it requires a little flexibility – is PICNIC. It is quite an appropriate acronym for Social Action Research as, by strict definition, a picnic is not just a meal that one eats outdoors, but a meal in which all the participants bring something to contribute to the collective experience of eating together.

Participatory	Facilitates the full involvement of research subjects and other stakeholders in all stages of the research.
Inductive	Draws theory out of data rather than interprets data and organises data within predefined or given frameworks.
Critical	Grounded on a power perspective, committed to social change to the advantage of those currently without power.
aNti-oppressive	Actively challenges assumptions which underpin unequal social relations, with an explicit commitment to empowerment and social justice.
Iterative	Builds up theory and knowledge progressively.

Cyclical   A process that continually revisits and evaluates its build-
                  ing blocks.

Social Action Research in practice

We now offer an example of what the theory set out above looks like in
practice. The concepts and ideas are the backdrop to the research we
develop in practice. Social Action Researchers look for opportunities to
maximise all the principles and philosophies in the practice of research – to
maximise people's involvement and participation throughout every piece of
work. The example we offer is that of a community consultation about play
and childcare facilities in Nottingham, called the Child Care Research
Project.

The Child Care Research Project

Social Action Research methodology usually falls into a number of main
phases. These are not separate and discrete, but will overlap between stages.
On this occasion there were eight phases:

- orientation phase and review of written materials;
- establishing a research steering group;
- recruiting and training local people as information gatherers;
- establishing the parameters of the research and appropriate methods
  for information collection;
- gathering the data;
- analysing the data through further consultation;
- preparing and presenting a final report;
- dissemination of, and action on, the research findings.

A local group was established by the City Council Area Committee to
develop training, education and employment opportunities in the locale
covered by the committee. Members included local community and statutory organisations' representatives already working on these issues (such as
health visitors, representatives from the local FE college, tenants' and residents' associations, play workers, voluntary groups promoting play in the
area, community workers and youth workers). Discussions at the group
meetings focused on identifying barriers to take up of training and education and employment opportunities already in existence in the area. The
group considered lack of affordable and quality childcare as the main
obstacle. In addition, they were aware that whilst there was very little registered local childcare, there were a lot of informal arrangements. This led
them to ask a number of questions: 'Are people happy with informal
arrangements?' 'What other provision would parents and children like to

see?' 'Why do so few childminders in the area register and what kind of support would they find useful?'

The Centre for Social Action was approached by the local group and, in partnership, the two organisations made a successful funding application to the Health Action Zone to carry out a research project investigating childcare needs among local communities and collecting views and experiences from parents and children. A broad definition of 'childcare' was used, from play through to places where parents could leave children while they went to work.

Both the Centre and the Local Steering Group wanted to employ local people to be the researchers and gather the information on this project and intended that these people should be very active in developing the parameters of the research. There were a number of reasons for this. It was felt that to use local skills and knowledge was important. The area consisted of communities that were quite closed – difficult for outsiders to enter. There was considerable local resentment regarding outsiders employed and paid to work in the area leaving at the end of each day to spend their salaries elsewhere. Hence, it was very important that local people were seen to be integral to the whole of the research process. Employing locals as researchers also offered an opportunity for local skill development. Most importantly, it was an opportunity to put money into the community. The budget included reasonable rates of pay for people to undertake the research and to attend training and support meetings.

Originally it was intended that the project should be locally managed, and have local responsibility for the financial management and payment of workers. However, to meet the funder's governance requirements it was necessary for De Montfort University to manage the project. This led to a number of problems, most particularly delays remunerating the people involved. Nevertheless, the project was directed by people who lived and worked in the area and who were well placed to continue the community process by taking action on the findings of community consultation. One of the authors took the role of 'research advisor' and worked closely with local people in all aspects of the project.

Recruitment and employment

A local woman (single parent) was recruited as coordinator, administrator and local point of contact for the project. She disseminated initial publicity, creating flyers, posters, information leaflets and letters to organisations in the community. She was also involved in radio and local press interviews in order that local people and organisations knew about and could become interested in the project. It was also necessary to inform residents that the project wanted researchers. As a result, approximately 20 people responded.

The Steering Group developed a person specification and job description for the researchers (set out in Boxes 9.1 and 9.2). The person specification included aspects of being able to work on one's own, being a good listener and learning new skills. However, the Steering Group considered that experience of childcare was an important criterion and wanted to be open as to what they considered to be childcare experience (to include being a parent, a childcare worker, a babysitter or someone looking after other family members). They also specified that they were looking for people who spoke community languages and that there would be better remuneration for those conducting interviews in community languages but reporting in English.

People who expressed an interest were sent these materials and an application form. Twelve people formally applied and were invited to a selection

---

Box 9.1 Researcher's person specification

- be able to work as part of a team;
- have a friendly and approachable manner;
- be able to encourage people to voice their views and opinions;
- be a good listener;
- be enthusiastic and willing to learn new skills;
- be able to work on own initiative;
- have a reasonable level of literacy;
- display experience of childcare through being a parent or a childcare worker, including babysitting and looking after family members
- be able to work with groups of parents and children;
- be reliable and trustworthy;
- pass satisfactory police check.

Box 9.2 Researcher's job description

- attend the training and support sessions;
- arrange own interviews with groups, organisations and individuals as agreed;
- use agreed format for facilitating group and individual conversations with parents and/or children;
- produce adequate written records of all discussions and interviews;
- be responsible to project coordinator and research advisor.

morning with a dual purpose: to enable them to find out more about the project and to create a safe, comfortable environment in which they could show what they had to offer the project. There were a series of activities including interviewing each other, a groupwork exercise designing a poster for the project (which was subsequently used), considering the pros and cons of different methods of information collection and writing a report of the morning. These gave some idea about whether people felt competent to take part in the project and highlighted their observational and written skills. All twelve people were considered suitable to be researchers but only eight expressed an interest in the position. The major reason for people not wanting to continue was the difficulty of short-term employment whilst claiming benefits.

On the selection day, participants also listed the things they thought they would need to know in order to undertake the project. This was used in conjunction with previous research experience and the ideas of the Steering Group to create a training plan.

Training programme

Training took place over three separate days, one a week for three weeks, and identified a wide range of topics (see Box 9.3 for a full list). Training considered the qualities required to be a researcher, plus the areas of confidentiality and child protection. Understandably, people were concerned about what they should do if they saw or heard about a child at risk and, though the situation never occurred, they felt it important to be prepared. The sessions covered listening skills and interviewing children and were experiential, giving people the opportunity to practise skills and techniques they had learnt.

In both the Steering Group and researcher group, consideration was given to the topics to be explored, who to include and where and how contacts might be made. Both groups created a list of issues around the subject of childcare and play in the area, which were grouped and themed, and the researchers tried out ways of asking questions that would elicit information about the topics and issues. It might have been tempting to develop a long questionnaire with closed answers to ensure all topics were addressed but this would not fit with Social Action Research. Instead, a set of carefully worded open questions was created, piloted and refined many times, to enable respondents to present their perspective based on their own experience.

The researchers had to provide two references and complete a police check before they were able to make contact with people.

Ways of collecting data

The researchers, alongside the local Steering Group, decided on five ways of collecting information:

Box 9.3 List of topic areas for training purposes

Purpose of the research
Qualities needed to be good information gatherers
Confidentiality
Appearance and reliability
Safety
Child protection
Asking questions
Listening skills, probing and getting deeper answers
Interviewing children
Group interviews
Recording
Issues that needed covering:
• What do we what to find out?
• Who should we ask?
• Where are good places to meet parents, young people and children?

• group interviews with children, aged from six years old upwards;
• group interviews with adults;
• long individual questionnaires for adults;
• long individual questionnaires for children and young people;
• short questionnaires for adults to be completed on the street, outside the school gate, in the park or at the post office.

The range of data collection methods encouraged a breadth and depth of information, reflecting people's community experiences. Time was spent on preparation, whereby researchers were confident about the new responsibilities. Researchers were keen to take the position seriously to illustrate people's views and opinions.

Ethics

Though ethical approval was not sought in this instance (at this time De Montfort University did not have an ethics committee for social work and community development research), ethical considerations are central to Social Action Research (see Fleming and Ward 1996) and were considered. All participants were told about the research and what would happen to the information, and verbal informed consent was obtained from everybody. In addition, issues of confidentiality and child protection were discussed in languages appropriate to the interviewee. Questionnaires were coded to preserve anonymity and, where conversations were taped, tapes were wiped clear once the information had been transferred to a recording sheet. The usual standards of research ethics were therefore maintained – 'permissions obtained, confidentiality maintained, identities protected' (Denscombe 1998: 63) – and it was considered that the research would have met the criteria of the Code of Ethics for Social Work and Social Care Research proposed by Butler (2002).

Remuneration

Remuneration was based on different activities undertaken. Researchers were paid a fee per interview, with different rates for group, individual and short interviews. The researcher group wished to work to the principle of equity. The principle was that everybody in the group would be able to earn the same amount of money and it was a principle that was very important to the group. Researchers agreed they would all do the same number of group interviews and individual in-depth interviews, though a number of people were not interested in doing the quick questionnaires on the street.

There were resources in the budget to cover childcare arrangements for researchers and parent group sessions. Though resources were only used for two researchers' children to go to the local playgroup, this was a big success with the children and they continued to use the playgroup after the research had finished. All group meetings were held in places where childcare was provided, with donations given to the service providers and voluntary organisations.

Support, access and liaison

The researchers were given tape recorders, pens, maps, questionnaires, time sheets, record sheets, claims forms, address lists and all the necessary paraphernalia to start data collection, and were supported on a weekly basis by the research coordinator who met with them at the local community centre café. Data were then returned or sent by post in pre-paid envelopes. It was surprising how many people actually came to the meeting place, dropping questionnaires off and having a cup of tea and a talk with each other about how things were going. The opportunity to meet and share experiences appeared to be very important. In addition, there were monthly meetings of all the researchers, the research coordinator and the research advisor, which researchers were expected to attend. At these meetings the process of information collection was discussed as was the need to contact a cross-section of the population including all key groups and organisations. If there were any difficulties, the research coordinator or advisor would undertake the initial contact which the researcher would then follow up. The content of what they were finding out was the focus of these meetings and so was at the heart of the analysis of information.

Personal contacts were crucial to access and researchers made enormous efforts to get into the community. There were refugees with families in the community, disabled children, disabled parents, homeless parents and parents who had themselves been in care. Researchers made considerable effort, through contacts, to collect a range of experience and it is clearly debatable whether, if the research had been conducted by a research academic, access would have been as successful.

The researchers spoke to a total of 514 people, of whom 375 were adults and 139 young people. The principle of equity soon became an issue, with some researchers working more quickly than others. Those completing data collection first were somewhat less patient and keen to take on more work. Maintaining these researchers' enthusiasm whilst waiting for others to complete their work was challenging. Those who took longer often had other commitments – were carers, had different life experiences or worked at a slower pace. The only researcher speaking any of the community languages left for Pakistan during the course of the project. Nevertheless, there was access to interpreters through an Asian women's project represented on the Steering Group.

Data analysis

Once the primary information collection was completed, it was time to commence data analysis. A whole-day meeting with the researchers led to a discussion of themes and identification of 'patterns and processes, commonalities and differences' (Miles and Huberman 1994: 9). There were a number of themes and approximately 30 initial coded categories, which were honed down through further analysis. Researchers were keen for categories to include the breadth of data collected. In some cases, there might be a particular experience, which one or two people had, but the researchers argued that these were still important experiences, and stressed the need to try and find some way of incorporating them into the findings.

The findings were a surprise to the Steering Group who, at the beginning of the project, had clear ideas about expected outcomes, for example, 'we need a toy library'. However, they were committed to finding out what local people thought and nobody from the community mentioned a toy library. Rather, they mentioned bigger things than expected, identifying broader issues such as the cost of provision, the condition of the parks and lack of support for parents. Some members were surprised at the local people taking a step back, highlighting more issue-based findings. Children and young people were not saying 'oh we want a swimming pool and an ice-skating rink', but places to go where they would not be bullied, parks where there was neither dog dirt nor syringes under swings. Respondents were realistic in what they wanted. Bullying and racism were big issues and flexibility was important. The needs of young parents, although they were a minority in the sample, were clearly defined. They felt there was little support for them outside the generic parenting services. A number of young parents had been in care and had no family support. Grandparents as carers was something that had not been considered prior to data collection, but as interviewers were approaching anyone with a child on the street, a number of grandparents were included in the respondent sample. Grandparents were seen to be fostering or having children living with them full time, and reported very little personal support.

Alongside the Steering Group, the research advisor produced an initial report in the form of a newsletter incorporating the views collected in themes agreed by the researchers. It set out what children and young people said, what adults said, what children and young people would like and what adults would like. It then set out 13 agreed themes and people were asked to rank the issues in priority order, first as personal opinion and second in terms of the community as a whole. This was a means of involving the wider community both in the analysis and the prioritisation of themes. It also gave people an opportunity to see where their experiences fitted the community experience. There was also room for free comment on the return slips.

Community response

Returns from the 400 newsletters disseminated showed racism and bullying as major issues for parents and children. There were comments such as 'whilst my family and myself have never experienced it, the report said that it was happening, so that's what has to be the number one community issue'. In this way local people made a contribution to the analysis.

It was intended also that there would be public meetings to discuss the findings and give people the opportunity to discuss with the Steering Group members the way forward. However, the first two meetings were poorly attended and felt to overlap with meetings to develop a bid for 'Sure Start'.

Action points arising from the project

The final report of the Child Care Research Project became an action plan, and the Local Steering Group became the Child Care Development Group. It increased the number of local people in its membership and took on board the action plan, working on a number of key issues. Other local groups also took up some of the issues voiced, for example, the cost of childcare and play provision which arose again and again. The local community centre applied for money to fund subsidised places for both their after-school club and their playgroup. Another issue that arose repeatedly highlighted parents' and children's reluctance to use parks due to the presence of alcoholics, syringes and a whole range of other things that did not make it conducive for people to play or meet there. This led to a clean-up campaign by the City Council, and a local group of parents applied for funding for what they called 'Play in the Parks'. They employed play workers to run after-school and holiday sessions to encourage children back into the parks. Thus, action points arising from the research have been taken forward to create change in the area.

The researcher perspective

As part of the reflective element of the Social Action process, the Centre for Social Action undertook an evaluation of the researcher perspective to find out what researchers thought about being involved in the project. The Centre employed an independent person to explore their views.

It was clear that people became involved in the project for a whole range of reasons, some because they were parents and thought childcare was a crucial issue, some because they wanted the money, and some because they had done research before and thought it would be interesting. Everybody had a clear understanding of their role and the expectations on them:

> It was about encouraging people in the community who were most affected by the issues we were looking at to make their views known, particularly people who did not normally do that.

They felt training had prepared them well for the project tasks, liked the practical elements of the project and appreciated the role they played in designing the project:

> We had an incredible amount of influence on the design of the research and it was important to be included. I really appreciated that part of the process.

There were a couple of people at the training stage who thought, 'you're from De Montfort University and you ought to know what you are talking about, so why are you asking us? You should be telling us what to do.' It took a while for everyone to realise that while De Montfort University did have things to contribute, so did the researchers and the Steering Group. However, by the end of the project, those most unsure at the outset were the most vocal supporters of the process.

The researchers thought it was crucial that they were local, as this helped them both make contacts and gain enough confidence to encourage others to participate. Overall it was considered a positive experience, encouraging learning about research and issues faced in childcare. There was also a tremendous increase in self-confidence, with people facilitating discussion groups and approaching strangers in the street who had never done so before.

Earlier in this chapter, we said that we viewed empowerment as having both individual and collective aspects. Both individual and collective empowerment came together in this research. At an individual level the research was a very important experience for people, but empowerment was also considered to have worked on a collective level for the wider community. People let their views be known about changes that were happening, whilst some people were actively involved in the process of change.

The researchers were impressed that the research methods worked so well and worked with very different types of people, from grandmothers through to 17-year-old parents, disabled 11-year-olds through to Asian women using interpreters.

The researchers highlighted the importance of the flexibility of the research advisor and the fact that they were allowed to work at different paces, which suited their personal circumstances.

Inevitably, there were a few organisational and practical concerns. The major complaint was about having to wait to be paid. Delays were considered a failing of the project, though it is likely that De Montfort University is not alone in being slow to pay project members. However, alongside the 'benefits' issues, these need to be major considerations when employing local people on short-term contracts.

It was suggested that we should have recruited more than one Asian language speaker and, though the project did have access to interpreters, this was also considered a weakness. In addition, researchers suggested that they should have had more support. They did appreciate the weekly and monthly meetings but still felt that they could have done with more contact with the project team.

Finally, some of the researchers would have liked the training they received to have been accredited. Though they all received a certificate of attendance from De Montfort University, it was not an accreditation. The Steering Group looked into accreditation, but within the timescale of the project, it did not appear feasible, though it is reasonable to suggest that people who have put that amount of time and effort into training and research should be able to get an accreditation.

Conclusions

Social Action claims to offer an easy-to-understand, open-ended process. It enables people to identify and act on issues they deem important and work in any setting with any age group, and allows for a full consideration of relevant issues and problems before action is taken. It offers people the opportunity to act for themselves, outside pre-set programmes or initiatives, to transmit their views on matters that affect them directly and equip themselves with skills and expertise which continue to be positive assets long after their involvement in the project has ended. We hope the example offered shows how this can really be done in practice.

Social Action Research works in a spirit of enquiry, debate and discussion. It is not a tied-up and finished product, but a process of constant review and reflection. Social Action Research, as we hope is apparent from this chapter, involves planning, acting, reflecting and re-planning. It is a continuous cycle of learning from experience, a cycle which is fluid, open and responsive and also prepared to learn from the experiences of others.

Acknowledgements

This research project depended on the work and commitment of many people. It is important to acknowledge the work of the coordinator and the researchers and members of the Steering Group; also, of course, the community members – children, young people and adults – who took part in the research and contributed their views and opinions.

References

Ahmed, B. (1990) *Black Perspectives in Social Work*, Birmingham: Venture Press.
Baistow, K. (1994) 'Liberation or regulation?', *Critical Social Policy,* 42: 34–47.
Beresford, P. (2000) 'Services users' knowledge and social work theory: Conflict or collaboration?', *British Journal of Social Work,* 30: 489–503.
Beresford, P. and Evans, C. (1999) 'Research and empowerment', *British Journal of Social Work,* 29: 671–7.
Braye, S. and Preston-Shoot, M. (1995) *Empowering Practice in Social Care,* Buckingham: Open University Press.
Breton, M. (1994) 'On the meaning of empowerment and empowerment orientated social work practice', *Social Work with Groups,* 17, 3: 23–37.
Butler, I. (2002) 'Critical commentary (a code of ethics for social work and social care research)', *British Journal of Social Work,* 32, 2: 239–49.
Cress-Wesling, F. (1991) *The ISIS Papers*, Chicago: Third World Press.
Denscombe, M. (1998) *The Good Research Guide for Small Scale Research Projects*, Buckingham: Open University Press.
Dominelli, L. and McLeod, E. (1989) *Feminist Social Work*, London: Butterworth.
Fitzpatrick, S., Hastings, A. and Kintrea, K. (1999) 'Young people's participation in urban regeneration', *Child Right,* 154: 11–12.
Fleming, J. (2000) 'Action research for the development of children's services in Ukraine', in Kemshall, K. and Littlechild, R., eds, *User Involvement and Participation in Social Care – Research Informing Practice*, London: Jessica Kingsley.
Fleming, J. and Ward, D. (1996) 'The ethics of community health needs assessment: Searching for a participant centred approach', in Parker, M., ed., *Ethics and Community*, Preston: University of Central Lancashire, Centre for Professional Ethics.

Fleming, J. and Ward, D. (1999) 'Researcher as empowerment: The Social Action approach', in Shera, W. and Wells, L., eds, *Empowerment Practice in Social Work*, Toronto: Canadian Scholars' Press.

Foucault, M. (1980) *Power, Knowledge: Selected Interviews and Other Writings*, New York: Pantheon.

Freire, P. (1970) *Pedagogy of the Oppressed*, Harmondsworth: Penguin.

Gilroy, P. (1987) *There Ain't no Black in the Union Jack*, London: Hutchinson.

hooks, b. (1992) *Ain't I a Woman: Black Women and Feminism*, London: Pluto Press.

Hudson, A. (1989) 'Changing perspectives: Feminism, youth and social work', in Langan, M. and Lee, P., eds, *Radical Social Work Today*, London: Unwin Hyman.

Kemshall, H. and Littlechild, R., eds, (2000) *User Involvement and Participation in Social Care*, London: Jessica Kingsley.

Langan, M. and Day, L., eds, (1992) *Women, Oppression and Social Work*, London: Routledge.

Lorde, A. (1984) *Sister Outsider*, Freedom, CA: The Crossing Press.

Lukes, S. (1974) *Power: A Radical View*, Basingstoke: Macmillan.

Miles, M. and Huberman, M. (1994) *Qualitative Data Analysis*, 2nd edn, London: Sage Publications.

Morris, J. (1998) *Don't Leave Us Out – Involving Disabled Children and Young People with Communication Impairments*, York: Joseph Rowntree Foundation.

Mullender, A. and Ward, D. (1991) *Self-Directed Groupwork: Users Take Action for Empowerment*, London: Whiting and Birch.

Oliver, M. (1990) *The Politics of Disablement*, Basingstoke: Macmillan.

Page, R. (1992) 'Empowerment, oppression and beyond: A coherent strategy? A reply to Ward and Mullender', *Critical Social Policy*, 35: 89–93.

Shaw, I. (2000) 'Just inquiry? Research and evaluation for service users', in Kemshall, H. and Littlechild, R., eds, *User Involvement and Participation in Social Care*, London: Jessica Kingsley.

Staples, L. (1990) 'Powerful ideas about empowerment', *Administration in Social Work*, 14, 2: 29–41.

Staub-Bernisconi, S. (1991) 'Social action, empowerment and social work – an integrative theoretical framework for social work and social work with groups', in Vinik, A. and Levin, M., eds, *Social Action in Group Work*, Binghampton, New York: Haworth Press.

Thomas, M. and Pierson, J. (1995) *Dictionary of Social Work*, London: Collins.

Ward, D. (2000) 'Totem not token: Groupwork as a vehicle for user participation', in Kemshall, K. and Littlechild, R., eds, *User Involvement and Participation in Social Care – Research Informing Practice*, London: Jessica Kingsley.

Ward, L. (1997) *Seen and Heard: Involving Disabled Children and Young People in Research and Development Projects*, York: Joseph Rowntree Foundation.

Willow, C. (2002) *Participation in Practice: Children and Young People as Partners in Change*, London: The Children's Society.

Wilson, A. and Beresford, P. (2000) 'Anti-oppressive practice: Emancipation or appropriation?', *British Journal of Social Work*, 30: 553–73.

Zarb, G. (1992) 'On the road to Damascus: First steps towards changing the relations of disability research production', *Disability, Handicap and Society*, 7, 2: 125–38.

Index

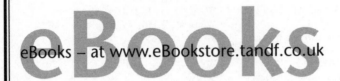